Charles Seale-Hayne Library
University of Plymouth
(01752) 588 588
LibraryandITenquiries@plymouth.ac.uk

Coming of Age

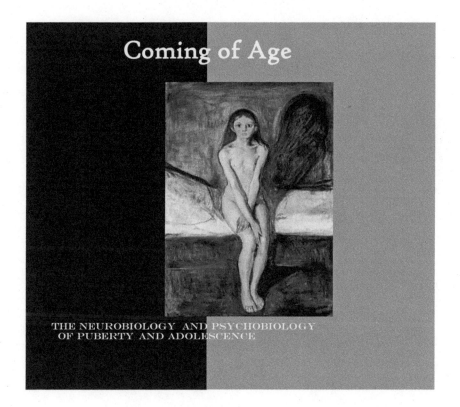

Coming of Age

THE NEUROBIOLOGY AND PSYCHOBIOLOGY
OF PUBERTY AND ADOLESCENCE

Coming of Age

The Neurobiology and Psychobiology of Puberty and Adolescence

CHERYL L. SISK

RUSSELL D. ROMEO

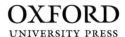

OXFORD

UNIVERSITY PRESS

OXFORD
UNIVERSITY PRESS

Oxford University Press is a department of the University of Oxford. It furthers
the University's objective of excellence in research, scholarship, and education
by publishing worldwide. Oxford is a registered trade mark of Oxford University
Press in the UK and certain other countries.

Published in the United States of America by Oxford University Press
198 Madison Avenue, New York, NY 10016, United States of America.

CIP data is on file at the Library of Congress
ISBN 978–0–19–531437–3

1 3 5 7 9 8 6 4 2

Printed by Integrated Books International, United States of America

For my mom Nancy
C. L. S.

For Mary and Sophie
R. D. R.

Contents

Preface

The chances are pretty good that anyone reading this book will have already experienced puberty and adolescence and therefore will have first-hand knowledge of the considerable physical and behavioral transformations that occur during roughly the second decade of life. Most of us pull through this scary rollercoaster ride just fine, despite ourselves. In fact, adolescence is such a normal part of our experience that it is easy to take for granted the extreme makeover of our bodies and brains. If you think about it, however, this transition from childhood to adulthood is nothing short of a metamorphosis, during which various body parts are transformed to serve new functions.

The purpose of this book is to explore the neurobiology and psychobiology underlying puberty and adolescence. Specifically, we will trace how contemporary neuroscience has come to make significant contributions to the understanding of a developmental period that used to be the sole purview of developmental psychologists and pediatric endocrinologists. To be sure, many aspects of puberty and adolescence are still in the discovery stage of investigation. Although phenomena are still being described and a mechanistic understanding of them is still in the future, major advances have been made over the past 30 years, and the adolescent brain is much less of a black box now than it used to be.

We hope this book is provocative and challenging for those who are trying to grapple with and unlock the biological and psychological mysteries that are puberty and adolescence. While writing this book, we assumed the reader would have a general understanding of the basic principles of neuroscience and psychology and, as such, feel it would best serve as an appropriate text for an upper-level undergraduate seminar or graduate course designed to probe puberty and adolescence more deeply from a psychobiological perspective. With all of these assumptions in mind, we have attempted to write accurately, critically, and analytically about what we think are the most important aspects of the science, using a conversational style. At the end of each chapter, we refer the interested reader to in-depth reviews of specialized topics. We hope all will find our book to be an enjoyable read and welcome your comments and feedback.

Acknowledgments

"Hold your head up – you've been elevated to the awkward age of adolescence. This is the time when we feel unworthy, lonely and unfulfilled, and also the time to receive and to express ourselves, to liberate ourselves from the mediocre acts of carbon copying someone else. We are in a maze, staring at the skylights of beaming glass, moving forward and looking beyond the blank, empty walls and abstract skylights." Artist's reflection on "Adolescence—The Inevitable Maze". Original cover art by Alexandra Nechita, 2009.

We would like to thank Drs. Monique Ernst (National Institute of Mental Health), Megan Herting (University of Southern California), and Mary Vernov (Weill Cornell Medicine) for comments on earlier drafts of specific chapters. We would also like to thank an anonymous reviewer, as well as Drs. Ruth Wood (University of Southern California) and Linda Wilbrecht (University of California–Berkeley) for their thoughtful comments on the entire manuscript. Any factual or typographical errors in the text are our own, however.

We would like to thank the students in our laboratories over the years for their input, critiques, and suggestions on various chapter parts; in particular, Eman Ahmed, Margaret Bell, Kayla De Lorme, Jenny Kim, Sarah Meerts, Nancy Michael, Margaret Mohr, Heather Molenda-Figueira, Kaliris Salas-Ramirez, Kalynn Schulz, Elaine Sinclair, and Julia Zehr. We would also like to thank the Markus Library at Rockefeller University and Finnegan's Wake Pub for providing a welcoming environment conducive to working on this manuscript on the occasions away from our office.

We give special thanks and acknowledgments to Drs. Douglas Foster (University of Michigan) and Ruth Wood (University of Southern California) for our research collaborations and many stimulating discussions that provided the initial inspiration for writing this book.

Finally, we are indebted to our editor, Joan Bossert, for her extraordinary patience and support as we wrote this book. We couldn't have done this without her guidance and advice, and we are grateful for her encouragement at all stages. Thank you for hanging in there with us.

Coming of Age

1
Introduction

Puberty has been traditionally associated with hormonal changes that result in the appearance of secondary sex characteristics and reproductive fertility. For many years, these hormonal changes were blamed for the poor judgment and emotional volatility that often characterize adolescence—the commonly used "raging hormones" explanation of teen behavior. However, researchers now appreciate that puberty also marks the beginning of a period of extensive brain development and remodeling that spans adolescence and extends well beyond the age of reproductive maturity. For example, cortical areas involved in decision-making and emotional regulation are not fully mature until the 20s (see Chapters 4 and 5 for the full story on this topic). These recent discoveries have pushed the pendulum in the opposite direction, and capricious teen behavior is now more likely to be blamed on a "haywire brain." This book is written from the perspective that neither raging hormones nor a haywire brain in isolation accounts for adolescent behavior. Rather, it is the *interaction* between hormonal changes and brain maturation, coupled with changes in the quality of social interactions, that make adolescent behavior seem so unpredictable. We take the point of view that puberty and adolescence are separable, but inextricably linked developmental processes: The brain initiates puberty, and, in turn, the adolescent brain is a target of both pubertal hormones and experiences resulting from the changes that hormones cause in the body and brain.

To introduce our topic, and the remaining chapters of this book, let's start with operational definitions of puberty and adolescence, terms that are sometimes used interchangeably and synonymously. We define puberty as the process of becoming capable of sexual reproduction. We define adolescence as the transitional period from childhood to adulthood. Adolescence therefore encompasses puberty but extends well beyond purely reproductive maturation to include the development of cognitive, emotional, and social behaviors that we associate with adulthood, behaviors that ultimately enable us to fend for ourselves and perhaps offspring as well. Also, if we acknowledge that sexual reproduction usually requires complex social behaviors for bringing sperm and egg together, then the distinction between puberty and adolescence is again blurred. Fundamentally, however, puberty is about physiological and reproductive maturation, and adolescence is about neurobehavioral maturation.

Puberty and adolescence have been the subjects of scientific investigation for decades, although largely examined somewhat separately. For instance, puberty has been the focus of pediatric endocrinologists treating disorders of pubertal timing, such as precocious or delayed puberty, while adolescence has been the focus of developmental psychologists, who long recognized this period as a pivotal stage of cognitive and emotional maturation. Ironically, even though both puberty and adolescence obviously involve changes in the brain at a particular time in development—changes that transform the individual forever—neither puberty nor adolescence was within the purview of developmental neurobiology until relatively recently. But research on puberty, adolescence, developmental psychology, and developmental neurobiology is now gradually coming together, and no doubt this convergence will inform scientists working in each of these different fields.

As a case in point, we can trace the content of a series of international conferences, The Control of the Onset of Puberty. For over three decades, this conference periodically brought together clinical and basic researchers to discuss new findings on what governs the timing or "trigger" of puberty, the biological basis of the onset of puberty, and therapies used in the treatment of disorders of pubertal timing. The first four of these conferences, held in 1972, 1981, 1989, and 1994, were devoted exclusively to these topics, with virtually no mention of behavior or of any type of brain development not directly related to pubertal onset and maturation.

In 1994, the flavor of these conferences began to change, almost imperceptibly, with the gradual intrusion of the notions that (a) puberty is more like a process than an event, and (b) reproductive maturation requires not only endocrine and somatic development but also behavioral development. Consideration of behavioral maturation during puberty necessarily broadened the scope of the meetings to include additional social and cognitive behaviors associated with adolescence and the more globally occurring changes in the adolescent brain. By the fifth conference in 1999, scientific content expanded for the first time to include behavioral aspects of puberty. For example, there were presentations on the relationship between the pubertal increase in gonadal hormones and expression of sexual and aggressive behavior. There was even a presentation on adolescent-related refinements in prefrontal cortex circuitry and the relationship to schizophrenia, a disorder that mainly becomes manifest during late adolescence (Lewis, 2000). The final meeting in this series, held in 2005, featured numerous talks on behavior and adolescent brain development (Giedd et al., 2006; Michaud, Suris, & Deppen, 2006; Schulz & Sisk, 2006), plus a provocative talk on the evolution of the age of puberty onset in humans in relation to societal and cultural expectations of teenagers (Gluckman & Hanson, 2006a).

Fueling this remarkable transformation in the scientific content of these and other conferences was the explosion of research reports in the decade spanning 1995 to 2005. Specifically, those published papers documented the profound spatial and temporal changes in the human brain across adolescent development (more on this in Chapter 4). Thus, by the beginning of the 21st century, puberty and adolescence made it into mainstream developmental neurobiology (Figure 1.1).

However, developmental neurobiology had some lessons to learn too. Less than 20 years ago, most neurobiologists would have agreed that as far as human nervous system development goes, all the heavy lifting is done during prenatal and early postnatal life, and by 5 years of age, the nervous system is pretty much a done deal. We thought this partly because brain size grows rapidly over the first few years of life and then plateaus at around 5 to 6 years of age (Dekaban & Sadowsky, 1978) and because major developmental milestones like walking and language are achieved by this time. However,

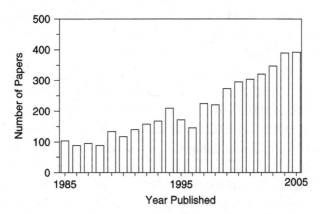

Figure 1.1. PubMed citations on adolescent and pubertal brain development from 1985 to 2005. Number of literature citations in PubMed per year (1985–2005) using these search terms: adolescence OR puberty AND human AND brain AND development.

thanks mainly to the arrival of magnetic resonance imaging (MRI), a noninvasive and safe way to image the brain, we have learned in the past 25 years that development of the nervous system is far from finished by 5 years of age. In fact, MRI has revealed a number of fascinating features of brain development during puberty and adolescence, including remodeling of the cortex, particularly in areas that manage decision-making, behavioral inhibition, regulation of emotions, and abstract reasoning. From this body of work, we now know that adolescent brain development extends well into the third decade of life.

As the imaging studies began to make their way into the scientific literature, fascination with adolescent brain development quickly spread beyond the research community. Many articles covering the "teen brain" have graced the covers, pages, and airwaves of *Time, New Scientist, Scientific American Mind and Brain, The New Yorker, National Geographic, The Wall Street Journal, Parade,* and National Public Radio, to name just a few. Popular explanations of irrational and impulsive teenage behavior in media formats such as these are now likely to include reference to the "immature" brain. In fact, recognition of the relative immaturity of the adolescent brain even surfaced in the judicial system (see Raeburn, 2004). In 1993, then 17-year-old Christopher Simmons was convicted of murdering a 46-year-old woman by pushing her car off a railroad bridge into a river. He was sentenced to death. In this landmark case, the Missouri Supreme Court overturned the death penalty sentence in 2003, and in 2004 the case went to the United States Supreme Court to decide on the constitutionality of the death penalty for individuals younger than 18 years of age. Based on MRI studies showing that the human prefrontal cortex is not fully mature until the early 20s, the defense before the Supreme Court questioned whether a 17-year-old brain is fully capable of impulse control and adult decision-making and reasoning, as these abilities are in part regulated by the prefrontal cortex. In effect, the defense was putting adolescence on legal par with developmental disabilities and, by extension, was arguing that moral culpability is not the same for adolescents and adults. The Supreme Court upheld the Missouri Supreme Court ruling and determined that the 8th Amendment (barring cruel or unusual punishment) and 14th Amendment (forbidding states to restrict basic rights) forbid the execution of offenders who are under 18 years of age when the crime is committed. Thus, based partially on neurobiological data on the adolescent brain, the Supreme Court ruled that a 17-year-old is considered to have significant limitations in reasoning, judgment, and impulse control and is therefore exempt from the death penalty (for more on this case and adolescent development of executive function, see Chapter 5).

The concept of the adolescent brain also resonates with people's own experiences. Jay Giedd, a pediatric psychiatrist and pioneer in using MRI to examine human adolescent brain development, and on whose work the arguments to the Supreme Court case were based, presented his research at the 2005 conference The Control of the Onset of Puberty. He began his presentation by telling the audience that whenever he mentioned to people that he was going to give a talk on the teen brain, this news elicited wisecracks like:

> "Short talk, huh?"
> "Oh, you mean they found one?"
> "What is your next talk on, the Loch Ness Monster?"
> "Isn't that a contradiction in terms?"

All jokes aside, there *is* a brain inside that adolescent body, and just as the body morphs during the second decade of life, the brain also undergoes an amazing transformation, the likes of which we are only beginning to appreciate.

As a final point in this introductory chapter, we want to say a little more about the relationship between puberty and adolescence. We have already distinguished the two physiologically and behaviorally by associating puberty strictly with reproductive maturation and associating adolescence with maturation of nonreproductive behaviors required for adult independence. Indeed, puberty and adolescence are separable, and as experiments of nature have shown us, we can have one without the other. Take precocious puberty in very young girls: If puberty is activated prematurely, say at 3 or 4 years of age, then ovarian and mammary gland development are initiated, but most people would not describe this process as adolescence. Cases like this are almost always treated quickly, so that premature ovarian development is halted. However, even if precocious puberty were allowed to proceed to fertility, few would refer to a fertile 4-year-old as an adolescent. The converse can happen too. Individuals with Kallman's syndrome, caused by the failure of specific neuroendocrine cells to migrate into the brain during embryonic development, do not go through puberty. However, they experience an adolescence in which they become adults in every sense of the word, except that they are infertile and, if untreated, do not have typical secondary sex characteristics. It is reasonable to argue that in these cases of delayed puberty, what appears to be adolescence is really an example of experience driving behavioral maturation. Similarly, even if a teenager is not going through puberty at the same time as their peers, they are nevertheless having (somewhat) similar social experiences, are subjected to the same set of expectations by parents and teachers, and are still going through a process that leads to personal independence, if not reproductive fertility.

On the other hand, as mentioned earlier, puberty and adolescence are intertwined, because they normally begin at more or less the same time and involve recurrent exchanges of signals and controls between the gonads and brain. That is, the hormones that rise during puberty shape the developmental trajectory of the organ that initiated puberty in the first place. The bottom line is that adolescence in the absence of puberty and puberty in the absence of adolescence are improbable and rare events, and in actuality, they are normally in alignment. Thus, perhaps a useful heuristic is to think of puberty as being a subset of early adolescence.

These interesting dissociations of puberty and adolescent timing in humans have led some basic scientists to explore this interaction using simpler and more experimentally accessible animal models. As an aside, it was not too long ago that some scientists questioned whether nonhuman mammals experience adolescence, on the premise that adolescence is a uniquely human experience. However, if the definition of adolescence is the physical and psychological transition from the juvenile state to adulthood and independence from caregivers, then, of course, nonhuman animals experience adolescence. With this supposition in mind, research with animal models, in which experience can be better controlled for and in which hormones can be manipulated independently of age, clearly tell us that some changes in the brain occur during adolescence even in the absence of pubertal hormones and unrelated to social experience during that time. Let us take as an example the developmental profile of expression of dopamine receptors in the neural "reward circuit" of the rat. In this circuit, dopamine-producing neurons in the ventral tegmental area (VTA) of the midbrain richly innervate the nucleus accumbens. When rats encounter or anticipate a reward, dopamine is released from the VTA nerve terminals and activates dopamine receptors present in neurons of the nucleus accumbens (for more on dopamine and reward, see Chapter 5). Using receptor binding as a proxy for receptor number, Susan Andersen and her colleagues mapped dopamine receptor binding in accumbens as a function of age in rats. They found an inverted U-shaped pattern, in which receptor levels increased during early adolescence and subsequently decreased during late adolescence (Teicher, Andersen, & Hostetter, 1995). Remarkably, however, this waxing and waning of dopamine receptors in the nucleus accumbens persists in rats that were castrated prior to puberty, thus demonstrating that the adolescent changes in dopamine receptor levels were not driven by pubertal changes in gonadal hormones (Andersen, Thompson, Krenzel, & Teicher, 2002). This, of course, begs the question as to what exactly is responsible for these seemingly spontaneous changes, but currently we simply don't know the answer.

As a decidedly less scientific example, those of us who have had pet male dogs may have noticed evidence for a behavioral change during adolescence that is not directly driven by pubertal hormones. We are referring to the sex difference in posture during urination that emerges during adolescent development in dogs. Prior to puberty, both female and male dogs squat to urinate, but as the dogs grow up, males begin to lift their legs and females continue to squat. It is tempting to attribute the change in posture in males to the influence of gonadal hormones during puberty. However, this change in urination posture occurs in male dogs that are neutered prior to the onset of puberty. Therefore, *something* must be happening in the brain during the normal time of adolescence that leads to this transformation of a fixed pattern of behavior in males.

The main point in all of this is that adolescent brain development is not simply "This is your brain on hormones." It appears that certain developmental changes in the adolescent brain are programmed to occur, with or without the influence of pubertal hormones. Nevertheless, when pubertal hormones are around, there is the potential for hormonal modulation of the developmental trajectory of the adolescent brain. Our overall perspective, then, is that the transition from childhood to adulthood that occurs during puberty and adolescence involves complex interactions between the developing brain, hormones, and experience. Change the timing or quality of any of these variables, and you have a different phenotype.

Our goal for the remaining chapters is to first try to dissect puberty from adolescent brain development and then put them back together again to show how they interact in various contexts. More specifically, Chapter 2 will review the neural mechanisms at the onset of puberty that activate the hypothalamic–pituitary–gonadal axis, the major neuroendocrine axis that controls gonadal hormone secretion. This chapter will cover when and how the brain knows to initiate puberty, such as we understand it today. Chapters 3 and 4 will cover the developmental neurobiology of adolescence.

These chapters will review the basic cellular mechanisms (Chapter 3) under-lying adolescent brain remodeling, including neurogenesis, programmed cell death, synapse formation and elimination (i.e., pruning), and myelination, and more global structural shaping of the adolescent brain along spatial and temporal continuums (Chapter 4). In Chapter 5, we begin to examine some of the cognitive changes that occur, in part because of this remodeling, and why some teenagers are prone to making some bad decisions. Chapter 6 will highlight how the pubertal rise in gonadal hormones interacts with the de-veloping adolescent brain and discuss how these hormonal changes program the expression of adult social behaviors, particularly those that are different between the sexes. Here we will also explore how the timing of puberty rel-ative to adolescent brain development affects the programming of adult be-havior. In Chapters 7 and 8, we examine the role of experience in adolescent development. In particular, we will explore how stress (Chapter 7) and drug use (Chapter 8) influence the adolescent brain. High levels of both stress and drug use are associated with human adolescence, at least as compared with other periods of life, and it is perhaps ironic that the adolescent brain appears more vulnerable than the adult brain to the adverse consequences of both stress and drugs. On the other hand, youth generally imparts more resilience, and we discuss whether the greater degree of plasticity inherent in the ado-lescent brain is an asset or a liability when experience is less than optimal. We will wrap things up in Chapter 9 by placing adolescent development in a lifespan context. Obviously, adolescence does not occur in a vacuum, and a cardinal rule of development is that what has happened earlier both sets the trajectory and limits the number of options for what can happen later. By this same token, what happens during adolescence constrains what can happen in adulthood. Interlaced in these discussions, we will frame what we believe are the most important remaining questions for basic research in puberty and adolescence from a psychobiological perspective.

Recommended Reading

Guyer, A. E., Silk, J. S., & Nelson, E. E. (2016). The neurobiology of the emotional adoles-cent: From the inside out. *Neuroscience and Biobehavioral Reviews, 70*, 74–85.

Herting, M. M., & Sowell, E. R. (2017). Puberty and structural brain development in humans. *Frontiers in Neuroendocrinology, 44*, 122–137.

Piekarski, D. J., Johnson, C. M., Boivin, J. R., Thomas, A. W., Lin, W. C., Delevich, K., . . . Wilbrecht, L. (2017). Does puberty mark a transition in sensitive periods for plasticity in the associative neocortex? *Brain Research, 1654*, 123–144.

2

Puberty

It Started With a Little Kiss . . .

It all started with a little kiss in 1996. Well, not exactly, and certainly not that romantically, but in the late 1990s cancer researchers at the Pennsylvania State University College of Medicine in Hershey, Pennsylvania, discovered a new gene. Remarkably, this gene, when expressed in a melanoma cell line, suppressed the process through which cancers spread. This finding provided scientists with a potential lead into halting the metastasis of certain cancers. This gene was given the name *KiSS-1*, as this "designation combines interim laboratory nomenclature for putative Suppressor Sequences with acknowledgment of the gene's discovery in Hershey" (Lee et al., 1996, p. 1733). A high honor for the little chocolate wrapped in foil. So how does the discovery of *KiSS-1* inform us about puberty? We will get to that shortly, but it turned out to be a missing link in an area of research far away from oncology.

A Primer on the Neuroendocrinology of the Hypothalamic–Pituitary–Gonadal Axis

Puberty onset is marked by substantial increases in hormones secreted by the hypothalamic–pituitary–gonadal (HPG) axis (Sisk & Foster, 2004). Similar to other neuroendocrine axes, the HPG axis works by releasing a domino-like cascade of hormones, the activation of which ultimately leads to the secretion of the gonadal "sex" hormones from the testes or ovaries, such as the androgens and estrogens. How the HPG axis functions is fairly well understood, but unraveling the mechanisms that get it started at the dawning of puberty is still a work-in-progress.

Although many of us are aware of the end products of the HPG axis, such as the steroid hormones testosterone and estradiol, less appreciated are the hormones produced "above the neck" that are ultimately responsible for the production and release of these gonadal steroids. The main player in all of this is a small peptide, only 10 amino acids long, called gonadotropin-releasing hormone (GnRH; occasionally referred to by its older name, luteinizing-hormone-releasing hormone or LHRH). Although small, this hormone is quite a big deal. In fact, after Drs. Roger Guillemin and Andrew Schally deciphered GnRH's structure, they were award the Nobel Prize in Physiology or Medicine in 1977 (sharing it with Dr. Rosalyn Sussman Yalow, who was instrumental in the development of radioimmunoassays, a widely used technique to measure hormone levels). GnRH is produced in neurosecretory cells loosely distributed throughout the forebrain. Although the exact distribution of these cells shows some species specificity, they are largely concentrated in regions of the hypothalamus, with the highest enrichment in the preoptic area in rodents, and the arcuate nucleus in primates (Baker, Dermody, & Reel, 1975; King, Anthony, Fitzgerald, & Stopa, 1985; Silverman, 1976). Independent of these differences between species, these relatively widely spaced GnRH neurons send their axonal projections to the median eminence at the base of the hypothalamus, emptying their GnRH payloads into the pituitary portal system. Once GnRH reaches the anterior pituitary gland, it binds to GnRH receptors on specialized gonadotropin cells, which, in turn, leads to the production and release of the gonadotropins, luteinizing hormone (LH) and follicle-stimulating hormone (FSH). These two hormones then enter the general circulation, journeying down to the gonads to induce the testes or ovaries to produce both the gonadal sex steroids and gametes (i.e., sperm and eggs), processes termed steroidogenesis and gametogenesis, respectively (Ojeda & Terasawa, 2002; Figure 2.1A).

In the context of gonadal steroidogenesis, the testes primarily secrete testosterone, while the ovaries produce mainly estradiol and progesterone. As these steroid hormone levels rise in the bloodstream, they act on the brain and pituitary gland to slow the release of GnRH and the gonadotropins, in effect reducing the flow of this hormonal cascade, a process termed negative feedback (Figure 2.1B). Negative feedback loops are standard operating procedures for neuroendocrine axes and are a common mechanism to maintain hormone levels at relatively steady concentrations (e.g., see Chapter 7 and our discussion of the axis that mediates the release of stress-related hormones). The "tone" of negative feedback is malleable, however, such that sometimes the HPG axis is more or less sensitive to gonadal steroids feeding back on the brain and pituitary. Indeed, the negative feedback brakes are really touchy prior to puberty and, in part, are responsible for keeping

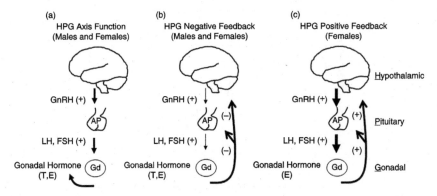

Figure 2.1. Structure and function of the hypothalamic–pituitary–gonadal (HPG) axis.
A simplified schematic of the HPG axis (a) as well as the negative (b) and positive (c) feedback properties exhibited by this axis. Note the thickness of the downward pointing arrows is associated with the decreased (thinner) or increased (thicker) drive to the anterior pituitary or gonad. AP = anterior pituitary; E = estradiol; FSH = follicle-stimulating hormone; Gd = gonad; GnRH = gonadotropin-releasing hormone; LH = luteinizing hormone; T = testosterone; (–) = negative feedback; and (+) = positive feedback.

the axis inhibited until puberty is ready to begin (Sisk & Foster, 2004; Sisk & Turek, 1983).

In addition to this sliding scale of negative feedback, the HPG axis has another trick up its sleeve, in that the axis can actually demonstrate positive feedback under certain conditions. In this case, as hormone levels rise in the bloodstream, the brain and pituitary gland start to release *greater* amounts of GnRH and the gonadotropins (Figure 2.1C). Positive feedback on the HPG axis is a rare occurrence, however. First, positive feedback occurs solely in females, at least under normal physiological conditions, and, second, this feed-forward situation happens only for a relatively brief period of time in a female's monthly menstrual cycle (or weekly estrus cycle in rodents), allowing for ovulation to ensue. It is the rising levels of estradiol released by the follicles in the ovaries that lead to a feed-forward–induced surge in LH and FSH, permitting the egg to be released. Thus, although this positive feedback phenomenon displayed by the HPG axis occurs infrequently, when it does, it turns out to be incredibly important for reproduction.

Prior to discussing the signals that direct the axis to start pumping out the previously mentioned hormones at the onset of puberty, one more

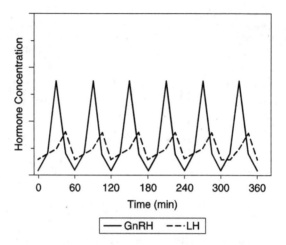

Figure 2.2. Pulsatile release of gonadotropin-releasing hormone (GnRH) and luteinizing hormone (LH).
GnRH and LH are released in a pulsatile manner with GnRH pulses stimulating the episodic release of LH. GnRH levels are represented by the solid line, and LH levels are represented by the dashed line.

notable parameter concerning HPG function should be noted, namely that the hormones secreted by the hypothalamus and the pituitary are released in a pulsatile, or episodic, manner. More specifically, if you were to measure GnRH and LH levels on an hourly basis in adult animals, you would see regular intervals of hormonal peaks and valleys, with peaks in GnRH and the gonadotropins occurring in relative synchrony (Clarke & Cummins, 1982; Urbanski, Pickle, & Ramirez, 1988; Figure 2.2).

This pulsatile pattern of release doesn't just abruptly appear at the start of puberty. Instead, it happens gradually, such that the early stages of puberty are marked by occasional, low amplitude pluses, which are then followed in the later stages of puberty by pulses showing greater frequency and significantly higher peaks (Ojeda & Urbanski, 1994; Sisk, Richardson, Chappell, & Levine, 2001; Watanabe & Terasawa, 1989; Figure 2.3). It is important to note that the pulsatile nature of these hormones is not just for show, as there appears to be crucial information in the metronomic release of these hormones. For instance, if the pituitary gland is constantly exposed to high levels of GnRH, the gonadotropes are desensitized, resulting in drastically reduced LH secretion. In fact, and perhaps counterintuitively, this type of tonic exposure to GnRH can be used to inhibit the HPG axis in cases of precocious puberty,

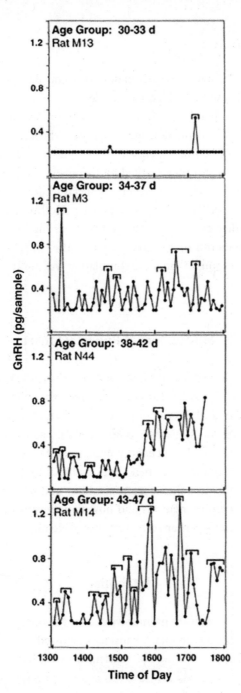

Figure 2.3. Pubertal development of gonadotropin-releasing hormone (GnRH) pulsatility.

The changes in GnRH pulse profiles in female rats during pubertal development. Note that as the animals age the frequency and amplitude of the GnRH pulses increase. Reprinted from C. L. Sisk, H. N. Richardson, P. E. Chappell, & L. E. Levine, 2001, In vivo gonadotropin-releasing hormone secretion in female rats during peripubertal development and on proestrus, *Endocrinology, 142,* 2929–2936. Used with permission from Oxford University Press.

when the axis is activated too early in development (Bhasin, Yuan, Steiner, & Swerdloff, 1987; Mann, Gould, & Collins, 1984).

If, on the other hand, GnRH is given in the more rhythmic, naturally occurring fashion, the gonadotropes respond with significant bursts of LH and FSH. Along these lines, men with idiopathic hypogonadotropic hypogonadism (IHH), a disorder marked by the absence of puberty caused by dysfunctional GnRH secretion, can be induced to undergo puberty if they are administered GnRH in a pulsatile pattern (Hoffman & Crowley, 1982). Thus, as with other biological systems, like signaling between neurons for example, it appears this on–off stimulation of the GnRH receptors leads to a more optimal response than if the stimulation was always stuck in the "on" position.

Modulators of Pubertal Onset

Now that we have introduced the hormones and the roles that they play in the function of the HPG axis, let's turn to what directs the production and release of these hormones at the onset of puberty in both ultimate and proximate contexts. Here, we will discuss how one's metabolic status ultimately informs the body that one has sufficient energy stores to sustain various reproductive functions, like pregnancy. We then shift our focus to the more proximate, cellular causes, including the neurotransmitters and neuropeptides that activate GnRH-containing neurons and how they permit the GnRH cells to follow the guide set by perhaps the most crucial element: gene networks.

Metabolism

Perhaps the most significant permissive cue for the onset of puberty is body weight. A seminal study in rats, for instance, showed that body weight, and not chronological age or "bone age" (skeletal growth), was the best predictor of pubertal onset (Kennedy & Mitra, 1963). They cleverly figured this out by providing rat pups with different amounts of postnatal feeding by manipulating the number of pups in the litter (i.e., fewer pups = greater chances of nursing = greater weight gain). Although animals were the same chronological and bone age at weaning, the "restricted" animals weighed half that of the "nonrestricted animals." These restricted animals went on to show a much later onset of puberty, as indexed by vaginal opening, estrus cyclicity, and mating, lagging behind their nonrestricted counterparts by almost a week (Kennedy & Mitra, 1963). Although studies in which nutrition is manipulated experimentally cannot be done ethically in boys and girls, similar results are found in that a critical body weight apparently needs to be achieved for pubertal processes to ensue in humans (Frisch & Revelle, 1970). The critical variable, however, is not body weight per se, but instead the level of body fat. It appears that, all other things being equal, the greater amount of body fat one possesses, the more likely the individual will experience the onset of puberty. This is particularly true in females, as the body needs sufficient energy stores to sustain a potential pregnancy, not to mention lactation (Kaplowitz, 2008). This may help explain why the age of pubertal onset continues to trend earlier in the developed world as obesity levels rise (Li et al., 2017; Wagner et al., 2012).

However, what is it about fat that informs the body that the internal metabolic environment would be conducive to puberty? The signal is a hormone released by the fat cells known as leptin. This hormone, so named for the Greek *leptos*, or thin, is encoded by the *ob* gene (ob for obese; Zhang et al., 1994). Leptin can have some rather dramatic effects on body weight and body fat (Friedman, 2016). For instance, mice that do not produce leptin, because of a mutation in the *ob* gene, show profound levels of obesity, an effect that can be completely reversed by exogenous administration of leptin (Pelleymounter et al., 1995). More germane to discussion here, however, is that leptin levels influence the timing of puberty. A study in young boys, for example, showed a significant relationship between circulating leptin levels and pubertal onset, such that serum leptin levels rose about 50% right before puberty was initiated (Mantzoros, Flier, & Rogol, 1997). A similar association between leptin and puberty was observed in girls, with higher leptin levels predicting an early age of menarche (Matkovic et al., 1997). These correlational studies would suggest that rising leptin levels might serve as a "trigger" for puberty. However, a correlation between two variables does not necessarily indicate causality, and this is where experimentally controlled animal studies have been helpful.

In the mid-to-late 1990s, a number of experiments conducted in male and female mice solidified the importance of leptin as a key player in the initiation of puberty. The first line of evidence is that normal mice administered leptin undergo puberty earlier than mice not treated with leptin (Ahima, Dushay, Flier, Prabakaran, & Flier, 1997; Chehab, Mounzih, Lu, &

Lim, 1997). The second line of evidence comes from the mice with the *ob* gene mutation. These mice are infertile, showing low circulating levels of HPG-related hormones, as well as reduced testis volumes and viable sperm in males and reduced uterine weights and ovarian dysfunctions in females. However, if these leptin deficient mice are treated with leptin, these neuroendocrine parameters and reproductive tissues come back online and begin to function properly (Barash et al., 1996).

These data indicate a clear effect of leptin as a permissive signal for puberty and reproduction function to commence. Less clear, however, is how leptin does this, and more specifically, how it affects the activity of the HPG axis. One conundrum is that GnRH cells do not express any appreciable level of receptors for leptin (Cunningham, Clifton, & Steiner, 1999). Instead, the actions of leptin appear to be through intermediaries, which, in turn, have direct actions on the GnRH cells. At this point, we need to come back to the *KiSS-1* story. As it turns out, signaling via *KiSS-1* serves as a go-between for leptin and GnRH activity (Castellano et al., 2009; De Bond & Smith, 2014; Smith, Acohido, Clifton, & Steiner, 2006; Wahab, Atika, Ullah, Shahab, & Behr, 2018) and, more broadly, was a missing link between many converging signals and the regulation of the HPG axis (Pineda, Aguilar, Pinilla, & Tena-Sempere, 2010).

Kisspeptin

Kisspeptin is the protein produced by the *KiSS-1* gene. As mentioned at the beginning of this chapter, this gene was known to play a role in the spread of certain cancers (Lee et al., 1996). However, its role in reproduction wasn't discovered until later, when two separate groups of researchers found that mutations in the kisspeptin receptor gene, *Kiss1r*, resulted in IHH, a disorder marked by the absence of puberty due to problems in GnRH function (Chevrier, Guimiot, & de Roux, 2011). Specifically, using a screen to find candidate genes that were associated with this disorder, it was found that individuals with IHH had a mutation in a gene called *GPR54*, and mice with targeted mutations of this gene had IHH (de Roux et al., 2003; Seminara et al., 2003). This gene encodes for a G-coupled protein receptor that recognizes a 54 amino acid ligand, hence the GPR54 alphanumeric. Prior to its discovery in the context of reproductive system function, GPR54 was known as an "orphan receptor," that is a receptor that shared the structure of other receptors with known ligands but did not have a known ligand itself. It turns out the

54 amino acid ligand for GPR54 is kisspeptin, and that is why the GPR54 receptor is also referred to as KiSS1r (r for receptor).

Kisspeptin is produced in neurons located in the hypothalamus, particularly within regions critically important in reproductive function, including the anteroventral periventricular nucleus (AVPV) and the arcuate nucleus (Clarkson, Han, Liu, Lee, & Herbison, 2010). These neurons send projections showing close apposition to GnRH cells, suggesting they release their kisspeptin cargo directly onto them. The GnRH cells also express GPR54. Moreover, if you chart the production of kisspeptin in the cells projecting to the GnRH cells, and the appearance of GPR54 on the GnRH neurons themselves, you see them rise prior to the onset of puberty and plateau later in adulthood (Clarkson et al., 2010; Figure 2.4). Thus, the signal and the

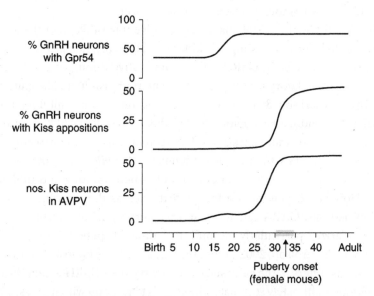

Figure 2.4. Pubertal development of kisspeptin- and GPR54-containing neurons. The temporal relationship between the percentage of gonadotropin-releasing hormone (GnRH) neurons with GPR54 (top trace), the percentage of GnRH neurons with close apposition to kisspeptin neurons (middle trace), and the number of kisspeptin neurons in the anteroventral periventricular nucleus (bottom trace) in the female mouse brain. Reprinted from J. Clarkson, S.-K. Han, X. Liu, K. Lee, & A. E. Herbison, 2010, Neurobiological mechanisms underlying kisspeptin activation of gonadotropin-releasing hormone (GnRH) neurons at puberty, *Molecular and Cellular Endocrinology, 324,* 45–50. Used with permission from Elsevier.

receptor appear to be in the right place at the right time to activate GnRH secretion to initiate puberty.

Kisspeptin, acting through the GPR54, causes GnRH neurons to depolarize and, hence, fire action potentials. Interestingly, one study reported that the number of GnRH neurons that respond to this depolarizing effect of kisspeptin increases during puberty, thus presumably leading to greater GnRH release (Han et al., 2005). Although it is still unclear what factors direct kisspeptin cells to "reach out" to GnRH cells prior to puberty—or, for that matter, what causes kisspeptin cells to increase their production of kisspeptin in the first place—it likely involves changes in the sensitivity of kisspeptin cells to gonadal hormones. However, this presents a "chicken and egg" question. That is, if gonadal hormones drive kisspeptin secretion, which drives GnRH secretion, which drives gonadal hormone secretion, then what gets this recursive process started in the first place?

Studies in female rodents have helped solve this riddle, and the answer turns out to be elegantly simple (Clarkson et al., 2010). It appears that prior to the onset of puberty, GnRH cells become active through a combination of increased excitatory inputs provided by neurotransmitters like glutamate or GABA (Clarkson & Herbison, 2006) and decreased inhibitory inputs mediated by endogenous opioids and GABA (Ojeda et al., 2006). For those of you with a little more background in neurochemistry, it may seem counterintuitive that GABA, the most ubiquitous *inhibitory* neurotransmitter in the nervous system, can do double duty—both exciting and inhibiting cells. However, depending on the context, such as the ion concentrations within neurons, GABA can act as an excitatory signal by causing neurons to depolarize, particularly around the time of pubertal onset (Han, Abraham, & Herbison, 2002). Once the GnRH cells are jumpstarted by these neurotransmitters in the early stages of puberty, then GnRH acting through the pituitary ultimately stimulates the gonads to respond with increased hormone secretion, which, in turn, feeds back up into the brain to activate the kisspeptin cells (Clarkson, Boon, Simpson, & Herbison, 2009). This activation now allows kisspeptin to take the wheel from glutamate and GABA and steer GnRH activity itself.

This working model is based largely on data from female mice. As such, many caveats need to be taken into account, including sex and species differences (Goodman & Lehman, 2012). However, even this nice, neat, and (relatively) straightforward account of GnRH cell activation and pubertal onset suffers from some missing elements. For instance, what gets the glutamate and GABA inputs going, what regulates the initial expression of glutamatergic and GABAergic receptors on GnRH neurons, and what signals the appropriate cells to synapse onto GnRH cells? Obviously, a simple "just because" will not suffice. So what is this *deus ex machina*? Genes.

Gene Networks and Puberty

The factors that regulate gene transcription are quite diverse and complex, but on a very simplistic level, gene expression can be activated or suppressed by signals originating from either inside or outside of the cell. These "autonomous" or "induced" changes in gene expression are what essentially dictate a cell's structure and function. It turns out that changes in gene expression play a fundamental role in initiating the early stages of puberty, which allow the previously described neuroendocrine changes to ensue (Ojeda, Lomniczi et al., 2010).

Many of the genes discovered to play a role in pubertal onset and timing were identified by using gene array analyses on hypothalamic tissue taken from experimental animals (e.g., monkeys and rats) in the peripubertal stages of development (Ojeda, Dubay et al., 2010). Gene arrays allow for the simultaneous measurement of the relative expression of many genes in a given tissue sample, so the simple idea was to see which genes showed substantial upregulation or downregulation during this stage of development in tissue where the majority of GnRH cells reside. These screens turned up many interesting suspects, many of which work as tumor suppressors in tissues outside of the brain and function relatively autonomously (Roth et al., 2007). These genes are arranged in a somewhat hierarchal fashion, such that lower tier genes responsible for proximate factors like glutamatergic and GABAergic functioning and kisspeptin signaling are controlled by the expression of higher tier genes, with alphanumeric designations such as *Oct2, Ttf1, Eap1, PcG,* and *Lin28b* (Ojeda, Dubay et al., 2010; Ojeda, Lomniczi et al., 2010). In essence, these "upper echelon" genes activate (e.g., *Oct2, Ttf1, Eap1*) or repress (e.g., *PcG* and *Lin28b*) the expression of the more proximate genes. These upper echelon genes, in turn, are controlled by myriad factors, including higher, higher tier genes, signals from inside and outside the cell, and epigenetic changes along these upper echelon genes themselves (Lomniczi et al., 2013; Roth et al., 2007). This polygenetic layering of genes may account for the variety of genetic deficits the have been reported to accelerate or delay puberty in human and nonhuman animals.

Epigenetic regulation of gene transcription and its influence on the expression of these genes are turning out to be a particularly interesting and important part of the puberty story (Lomniczi, Wright, & Ojeda, 2015; Messina et al., 2016; Rzecskowska, Hou, Wilson, & Palmert, 2014). Although the general term *epigenetics* means different things to different people, in this context, we are specifically talking about how epigenetic modifications of the DNA result in the silencing of genes through the process of methylation. DNA methylation occurs when a group of cytosine nucleotides of a gene becomes methylated by the action of DNA methyltransferase enzymes. This strip of methylation blocks the ability of transcription factors to bind to the DNA and do their job of transcribing. Conversely, demethylating these cytosines will permit transcription to occur. It was found that widespread disruption of DNA methylation, by the DNA methyltransferase inhibitor 5-azacytidine, or Aza, significantly delayed puberty in female rats (Lomniczi et al., 2013; Figure 2.5).

It may seem counterintuitive that increasing transcriptional activity blocks puberty, particularly if one thinks of puberty as an event that requires

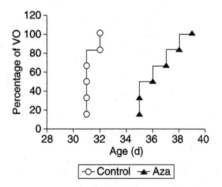

Figure 2.5. Delayed puberty following disruption of DNA methylation. The treatment of female mice with the inhibitor of DNA methylation, methyltransferase inhibitor 5-azacytidine (Aza; black triangles) delays their vaginal opening (VO), an index of pubertal onset. Note that all of the Aza-treated females show a later VO than all control-treated females. Reprinted from A. Lomniczi, A. Loche, J. M. Castellano, O. K. Ronnekleiv, M. Bosch, G. Kaidar, . . . S. R. Ojeda, 2013, Epigenetic control of female puberty, *Nature Neuroscience, 16,* 281–289. Used with permission from Springer Nature.

activation or "triggering." However, recall that genes like *PcG* and *Lin28* are actively repressing certain aspects of pubertal activation. Thus, one explanation of the previously described Aza result is that if the transcription of these repressor complexes is inhibited and the brakes on other "puberty genes" are released, then pubertal processes can proceed. For instance, one of the genes actively repressed is *Kiss-1* (Lomniczi et al., 2013). Under normal conditions, therefore, it would appear that epigenetic modifications of a set of repressor genes around the time of puberty, which results in their methylation, and hence silencing, permits the expression of genes that ultimately stimulate the activity of GnRH neurons.

As additional genetic and epigenetic factors are identified, this evolving story will undoubtedly become more complex. Moreover, at the very least, the signals that initiate the epigenetic modifications will need some clarification. One thing is for sure: the onset of puberty is the culmination of factors operating in exquisite balance, through a mixture of activation and inhibition, timing and tempo, and internal and external stimuli. However, would we expect anything less from a system that ultimately permits the propagation of our species?

Recommended Reading

Herbison, A. E. (2016). Control of puberty onset and fertility by gonadotropin-releasing hormone neurons. *Nature Reviews Endocrinology, 12,* 452–466.

Lomniczi, A., & Ojeda, S. R. (2016). The emerging role of epigenetics in the regulation of female puberty. *Endocrine Development, 29,* 1–16.

Manfredi-Lozano, M., Roa, J., & Tena-Sempere, M. (2018). Connecting metabolism and gonadal function: Novel central neuropeptide pathways involved in the metabolic control of puberty and fertility. *Frontiers in Neuroendocrinology, 48,* 37–49.

3

Remodeling the Adolescent Brain

What's in the Toolbox?

Now that we have introduced some of the fundamental parameters and processes that initiate puberty from a neuroendocrinological standpoint, let us turn to the remarkable structural remodeling that occurs in the nervous system during adolescence. In this chapter, we will start by looking at the underlying cellular mechanisms that are available to a developing nervous system and give examples of when and where these mechanisms are in play during adolescent brain maturation. In the next chapter, we will discuss the more global neuroanatomical changes that take place during adolescence as the results of these cellular processes.

House Remodeling and Gardening: Two Analogies for Neural Development

House Remodeling

In many respects, we can think about adolescent brain development in the same way that we think about remodeling a house: The foundation and structure are already there, and remodeling is for upgrades in functionality or for fine-tuning the inside organization of the house to accommodate new needs. To develop the analogy further, remodeling of a house might include expansion, which in the nervous system could amount to the addition of new cells or elaboration and outgrowth of neurites, such as axons and dendrites. Remodeling might involve turning a fledged child's bedroom into a parental hobby room, resulting in both a loss and gain of function. Upgrading the plumbing and fixtures in the bathroom is the equivalent of forming new neural connections and strengthening existing ones. Changing the motif of the living room from Victorian to American Southwest could be analogous to a developmental change in gene expression within a functional group of neurons. This brings us to a fundamental principle of nervous system development: There are only so many tools in the toolbox for construction and remodeling projects. A corollary to this principle is that the developmental processes that govern the initial wiring of neural circuits during fetal and perinatal maturation are used again when these circuits are rewired during puberty and adolescence. These tools and principle mechanisms of neural development and remodeling are, namely, cell proliferation, differentiation, migration, axon extension, synapse formation, cell death, and synapse elimination.

While we're talking about remodeling, now would be a good time to make the distinction between adolescent remodeling of the nervous system and what is conventionally meant by "neural plasticity." A simple way to view the difference between the two is to think of adolescent brain development as a fundamentally *proactive* change and neural plasticity as a fundamentally *reactive* change. Neural plasticity is an adaptive change in the structure and function of the nervous system as the result of experience. Learning the multiplication tables or a new language, practicing the piano or a tennis serve, and developing a taste aversion to tuna after a particularly nasty bout of food poisoning are all examples of neural plasticity. The operative word here is *adaptive*, meaning in response to or as the result of experience. In contrast, adolescent remodeling of the nervous system is a process that is *developmentally* programmed and timed—almost deliberate. This is not to say that experience does not matter during adolescence, because obviously it does. However, adolescent brain development is just meant to be—it is going to happen one way or the other—and experience is simply one variable that helps to sculpt the final product.

OK, then, so what times adolescent brain development? Chapter 2 was devoted to the external and internal triggers that time the onset of puberty, and even there we were left with question marks as to the nature of the developmental clock that provides gross timing of reproductive maturation. Unfortunately, we know even less about the developmental clock and permissive signals that time adolescent brain development. To us, this is one of the fascinating mysteries of adolescent brain development, and it might never really be solved. In fact, the question may even be inappropriate. For example, developmental biologists do not really ponder what times aging. It just happens, presumably through some process of genetic programming. Of course, endogenous and exogenous factors can speed it up or slow it down, or even lead to aberrations, but we are going to age whether we like it or not.

So for the purposes of this chapter, we'll take it for granted that adolescent brain remodeling is going to occur, and we'll focus attention on the factors that influence the developmental trajectory of the adolescent brain, and the fundamental mechanisms through which remodeling of the nervous system is accomplished.

Gardening

The house remodeling analogy is useful for thinking about certain building blocks and construction strategies involved in adolescent brain development, such as the addition of new cells or circuits or the rewiring of connections. These are processes that we can think of as progressive, which is defined as "moving forward or onward." However, nervous system development often involves events that can be thought of as regressive, or "characterized by increasing simplification of bodily structure." In the case of regressive events, gardening analogies are quite useful. One fundamental rule of nervous system development is to initially make more cells and connections than can be used or are needed and then to selectively eliminate those that either do not compete successfully for resources or that fail to thrive from lack of use. Every gardener knows this to be a good strategy at several points in plant development. Many seeds are sewn, and after germination, the seedlings are thinned for appropriate spacing according to the amount of resources available and the demands of the plant. Wayward branches are pruned to concentrate flower and fruit production in select branches that have better access to light or pollinating agents. It may feel wasteful to do these things, and sometimes it is difficult to accept that less can mean more, but it is all in the interest of producing strong, healthy, and efficient plants. The nervous system does the same things. For example, apoptosis, or programmed cell death, is commonly used to reduce the number of neurons that survive (Naruse & Keino, 1995). Synapse elimination is routine in the development of neuromuscular junctions (Sanes & Lichtman, 1999). Dendritic branches are initially elaborated and then selectively eliminated as male songbirds acquire their individual song (Nixdorf-Bergweiler, Wallhausser-Franke, & DeVoogd, 1995). In fact, neuroscientists have even adopted gardening terms for these developmental processes (e.g., synaptic or dendritic pruning, dendritic arborization, synaptic blooming).

House Remodeling and Gardening in Action

Developmental neurobiologists recognize at least four types of progressive and two types of regressive mechanisms used to construct the nervous system. These progressive events are (a) cell proliferation and differentiation, (b) cell migration, (c) axonal outgrowth and myelination, and (d) dendritic elaboration and synapse formation, and the two regressive events are (a) programmed cell death (apoptosis) and (b) synaptic pruning (synapse elimination). In this section, these progressive and regressive events will be described in more detail and examples of where they come into play during adolescent brain development will be given. Data in this section come largely, although not exclusively, from research using animal models.

Cell Proliferation and Differentiation

Stem cells in the central nervous system are both proliferative and multipotent. That is, they are capable of mitosis and of maturing into various cell types, including neurons and glia. Readers of a certain age may recall learning that mature neurons, unlike mature skin cells, for example, do not divide and replicate themselves, and therefore when they die, they are not replaced. These readers may also have been scared into thinking that because the vast majority of neurons are produced prenatally and because neurons don't self-replicate, then we humans are born with pretty much the entire complement of neurons that we're ever going to have, and from there on out it's all downhill in terms of numbers of nerve cells. We now know that this mid-20th century view of the nervous system wasn't entirely accurate, and it seems as though every decade since then has brought a new twist to the story of postnatal neurogenesis (Opendak & Gould, 2015).

It is true that mature neurons are not regenerative, in that they do not divide and replace themselves. But in the 1980s we learned that *adult* neurogenesis (i.e., the differentiation of proliferating precursor cells into neurons) occurs within the song system of adult canaries and other song birds that produce a new song each breeding season (Paton & Nottebohm, 1984). This shocking discovery not only meant that new neurons were predictably added to the adult avian brain, but that they must also somehow acquire the phenotype, connectivity, and functionality necessary for the production of a new song. While neuroscientists marveled at this revelation, there was still the presumption that adult neurogenesis was unique to birds. But, in fact, an early report in the 1960s foretold the phenomenon of adult neurogenesis in the mammalian brain (Altman, 1969). Using tritiated thymidine (^{3}H-thymidine), a method to label proliferating cells, neurobiologist Joseph Altman found that cells born in 30-day-old rats ended up in the olfactory bulb some 20 days later, and it was proposed that neurogenesis was a mechanism for renewal of the neuronal population in the adult olfactory bulb.

The neuroscience research community started to concede that neurogenesis did occur in the adult mammal, but—hold on—it is restricted to just a couple of privileged places where it makes sense to generate new cells. These "sensical" neurogenic regions were the subventricular zone, which gives rise to new neurons in the olfactory bulb (as Altman had suggested), and the subgranular zone, which gives rise to new neurons in the dentate gyrus of the hippocampal formation. These neurogenic neighborhoods made sense because the olfactory sensory neurons in the nasal epithelium turn over throughout the lifespan, so why shouldn't olfactory relay neurons in the olfactory bulb also do so? And wouldn't the addition of new neurons to the hippocampus be a perfect mechanism for the consolidation of new memories?

Once methods were devised to experimentally reduce neurogenesis, sure enough came solid evidence that newly added neurons to the olfactory bulbs and hippocampal formation do acquire function. Two methods commonly used to inhibit neurogenesis are targeted irradiation and antimitotic drugs that block cell division, such as methylazoxymethanol acetate (MAM) or cytosine arabinoside (AraC). Both head irradiation and systemic MAM treatment impair hippocampal-dependent types of learning (Leuner, Gould, & Shors, 2006; Shors et al., 2001). Similarly, it was found that infusion of AraC to the olfactory bulb causes female mice to lose their preference for a dominant male over a subordinate male, despite the fact that the AraC-treated mice can still discriminate odors (Mak et al., 2007). Thus, there is now general acceptance of the idea that adult neurogenesis in the hippocampus and olfactory bulbs contributes to functional plasticity in these brain regions.

Despite accumulating evidence to the contrary, there continued to be resistance to the notion that adult neurogenesis occurred in cerebral cortex and, even more so, the possibility that it occurred in phylogenetically older areas of the central nervous system. Slowly but surely, however, there has been an upward creep in the willingness to accept the phenomenon of adult neurogenesis in brain regions outside the subventricular and subgranular zones, and it is now well-established that new neurons are added in adulthood to the rodent amygdala (Fowler, Liu, Ouimet, & Wang, 2002) and hypothalamus (Chaker et al., 2016; Kokoeva, Yin, & Flier, 2005, 2007; Pierce & Xu, 2010; Robins et al., 2013). Furthermore, evidence is accumulating that new neurons in these brain regions are functionally integrated into neural circuits. The best evidence to date comes from labs studying adult neurogenesis in hypothalamic areas related to food intake and energy balance. For example, neurons added to the arcuate nucleus in adulthood appear to be involved in long-term regulation of body weight in adult rodents (Kokoeva et al., 2005; McNay, Briancon, Kokoeva, Maratos-Flier, & Flier, 2012; Pierce & Xu, 2010; Recabal, Caprile, & Garcia-Robles, 2017).

Well, OK, but what does *adult* neurogenesis have to do with puberty and adolescence? First, we can safely assume that postnatal neurogenesis is a potential mechanism for postnatal neuroplasticity. Second, if we accept the premise that the adolescent brain is being structurally and functionally remodeled, then what more interesting way to accomplish an extreme make-over than to bring in new leadership for a fresh look on life? Turns out there were hints of this dating back more than 25 years ago, had we been paying attention. In 1990, van Eerdenburg, Poot, Molenaar, van Leeuwen, and Swaab reported on the postnatal development of a newly identified oxytocin- and vasopressin-producing nucleus in the hypothalamus of the pig. They measured volume and neuron number in this nucleus at several postnatal time points and found that between birth and puberty more than 50% of the cells were lost. But beginning with the onset of puberty, there was an increase in the number of neurons, so that by young adulthood the number of neurons that had been seen soon after birth was not only restored but was exceeded (van Eerdenburg et al., 1990). Why didn't anyone jump on this finding? Who knows, but in the 1990s, adult neurogenesis in the hippocampus and olfactory bulb was just beginning to be accepted by mainstream neuroscience, adolescence was just emerging as a major period of brain development, and this was a cell group of unknown function in pigs. So, this paper just didn't make a splash, despite it having been published in the *Journal of Comparative Neurology*, known for its exacting standards and rigor in publishing neuro-anatomical papers.

As an aside, some years later, another research group reported that cells in this porcine nucleus highly express both proliferating cell nuclear antigen (PCNA), a cell proliferation marker (Rankin, Partlow, McCurdy, Giles, & Fisher, 2003), as well as oxytocin, suggesting that new cells making oxytocin are added to this nucleus during puberty (Raymond, Kucherapa,

Fisher, Halina, & Partlow, 2006). Given the roles of oxytocin and vasopressin in pubertally relevant functions, such as parturition, lactation, and social bonding (Benarroch, 2013; Bredewold & Veenema, 2018; Donaldson & Young, 2008), it's tempting to speculate these new cells in the hypothalamus are contributing to these important pubertal-related changes in a piglet's physiology and behavior.

Meanwhile, a laboratory in Spain was studying the development of a sexual dimorphism in the locus coeruleus (LC) of the rat. The LC is a group of mid-brain neurons that are the primary source of norepinephrine in the central nervous system. The adult female rat LC is larger in volume and has more neurons than the LC of the adult male rat (Guillamon, de Blas, & Segovia, 1988). This group discovered that this sex difference arose as the result of two postnatal periods during which growth of the female LC outpaced that of the male: the first two weeks of postnatal life and then again after the onset of puberty (Pinos et al., 2001). What is really interesting is that two different mechanisms seemed to be at play during these two periods. During the first 2 weeks of life, the number of LC neurons increased in both females and males, but there was also some apoptotic cell death going on, more so in males than in females. During the pubertal period, the number of LC neurons plateaued by 45 days of age in the males. In contrast, neurons continued to be added to the female LC between 45 and 60 days of age (Pinos et al., 2001). Based on these data, it's remarkable to think that neurogenesis during puberty actually leads to a substantial sex difference in a group of midbrain cells that influence virtually every circuit of the mammalian brain. However, these researchers did note that their data could also be explained by migration of much older, mature neurons from some other brain region into the LC (Pinos et al., 2001). The only way to tell would be to perform more sophisticated experiments, such as cell birthdating studies, which use nucleotides like thymidine that incorporate into and label dividing cells to track their fate, but so far this has not been done with the LC as a focus of study.

We have conducted cell birthdating studies to determine whether pubertal neurogenesis contributes to sex differences in hypothalamic and limbic regions of the brain. For these experiments, we used the thymidine analogue, BrdU, to label pubertally born cells in male and female rats and examined three brain regions known to show sex differences in adulthood (Ahmed et al., 2008). Two of these regions, the medial amygdala and the sexually dimorphic nucleus of the preoptic area (SDN) are male-biased (larger in males), and the other, the anteroventral periventricular nucleus (AVPV), is female-biased. BrdU was administered to rats that were at a prepubertal, early-pubertal, or mid-pubertal stage of development, and BrdU-labeled cells were examined 20 days later. Across all ages at which BrdU was administered, more BrdU cells were seen in the male medial amygdala and SDN than in the female, and more BrdU cells were seen in the female AVPV than in the male (Figure 3.1).

Similar to the ^{3}H-thymidine method used in the pioneering work done on neurogenesis, BrdU also labels dividing cells, but an additional advantage of the BrdU technique is the ability to phenotype the cells whose birthdate is known. That is, by double or triple labeling the BrdU positive cells via immunohistochemical methods, one can determine whether the cells are neuronal or glial and what transmitter substances, receptors, or other signaling molecules are present in the newly born cell. Double-labeling studies revealed that by the time these cells were 20 days old, some of them in the AVPV and medial amygdala had differentiated into neurons or glial cells. This finding was remarkable because it offered a novel mechanism, namely sex-dependent addition of new cells, for the establishment or maintenance of sexual dimorphisms in hypothalamic and limbic brain regions. Prior to this report, it was assumed that sexual dimorphisms were established during the perinatal period of development and passively maintained thereafter (the results of the Pinos et al., 2001, findings in the LC notwithstanding). So, now we have the possibility that new neurons are added to brain regions as a mechanism for enabling the brain to acquire the new functions that are necessary for the transition to adulthood. This is an especially enticing idea when the functions of these brain regions are considered. The medial amygdala interprets the meaning of social sensory stimuli, and everyone knows that social stimuli, such as interactions between friends (or potential mates), acquire new meaning during puberty and adolescence. The AVPV is headquarters for the generation of the preovulatory surge of luteinizing hormone (see Chapter 2), which is something that female rats can only do after puberty (and that male rats never do). So perhaps the recruitment of new neurons and glia is the brain's way of starting over or reassigning function during this developmental transition.

There was one more finding from this set of experiments worth mentioning here. If the rats were gonadectomized prior to puberty, effectively eliminating the pubertal rise in gonadal hormones, then the sex differences in pubertally added cells were completely eliminated (Ahmed et al., 2008). This raises the distinct possibility that pubertal hormones contribute to

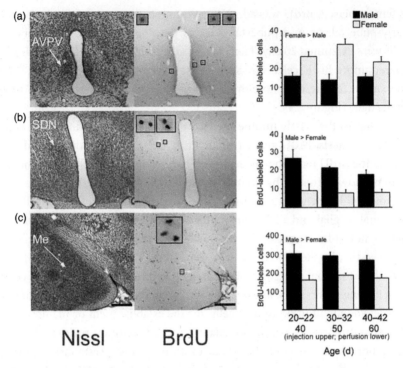

Figure 3.1. Neurogenesis in the adolescent rat brain.
Photomicrographs and data plots that show the pubertal-related addition of
new cells in the (a) anteroventral periventricular nucleus (AVPV), (b) sexually
dimorphic nucleus of the preoptic area (SDN), and (c) medial amygdala
(Me), nuclei relevant for male and female reproductive physiology and
behavior. Photomicrographs on the left are thionin-stained sections, while the
photomicrographs on the right are nearby BrdU-stained sections, as well as
insets with higher magnification photomicrographs of individually labeled cells.
The data indicate that females add significantly more cells to AVPV than males,
while males add more cells to the SDN and Me than females during puberty.
Scale bars in Panel C are 250μm. Reprinted from E. I. Ahmed, J. L. Zehr, K. M.
Schulz, B. H. Lorenz, L. L. DonCarlos, & C. L. Sisk, 2008, Pubertal hormones
modulate the addition of new cells to sexually dimorphic brain regions, *Nature
Neuroscience, 11,* 995–997. Used with permission from Springer Nature.

the remodeling of the adolescent brain by dictating when and where new
neurons and glia are added. As will be discussed in some detail in Chapter 6,
the presence or absence of gonadal hormones during adolescent brain development makes a big difference in how individuals behave in social situations,

and it seems likely that hormonal influences on neurogenesis and gliogenesis are an important part of that story.

Taking this a step further, one might predict that neurogenesis is a more prominent feature of the adolescent brain than the adult brain. In fact, Crews and colleagues (Crews, Mdzinarishvili, Kim, He, & Nixon, 2006; He & Crews, 2007) compared the number of new cells added to the olfactory bulb and dentate gyrus in adolescent and adult male mice and rats, and found that neurogenesis was significantly greater in adolescence than in adulthood. Other groups have similarly reported that cell proliferation in the hippocampus is higher in adolescent rodents compared to adults (Ho, Villacis, Svirsky, Foilb, & Romeo, 2012; Kim et al., 2004; Shome, Sultana, Siddiqui, & Romeo, 2018; Toth et al., 2008). From these observations, it is reasonable to deduce that the addition of new neurons is one mechanism by which the adolescent brain acquires new function. It also appears that the adolescent brain is more receptive than the adult brain to stimuli that promote cell proliferation. For example, some of the rats in the previously cited Kim et al. (2004) study ran on a treadmill for 30 minutes a day for 5 days. Here, exercise increased the number of proliferating cells in adolescent, young adult, and older adult rats compared to age-matched rats that did not run, but this effect of exercise was most pronounced in the adolescent rats. Even more surprising is the finding by Toth et al. (2008), also previously cited, that showed that chronic mild stress increases cell proliferation in adolescent rats, while the same experience decreases proliferation in adulthood (more on this in Chapter 7). Thus, the adolescent brain seems ready and willing to make new cells, and perhaps more so than the adult.

Nevertheless, that does not necessarily mean that the adolescent brain is a more hospitable place for those new cells to survive. For instance, in our experiments discussed previously about changes in neurogenesis in the AVPV, SDN, and medial amygdala, another group of rats was treated with BrdU either during adolescence or in adulthood, and brains were collected at either short (1 day) or long (30 days) survival times after BrdU treatment to assess cell proliferation and cell survival, respectively. Sure enough, the number of proliferating cells was higher in adolescent animals than in adults, no surprises there. What was surprising, however, was the number of cells that survived (and presumably went on to make a living somehow) was the same in adolescents and adults (Staffend, Mohr, DonCarlos, & Sisk, 2014). So, it would appear that by producing more new cells than the adult brain, the adolescent brain has more options to choose from in selecting which cells will stay and which will go.

Apoptosis

As previously described, the developing nervous system generates many more neurons than will actually stick around. Apoptosis, also known as programmed cell death, is an essential mechanism that removes excess cells and cells that do not successfully compete for spots in the developing organ. It is important to note that apoptosis is a special type of cell death and is different from necrotic cell death resulting from injury, disease, or toxicity. The cellular events that underlie apoptosis have been pretty well worked out. The short story is that there are families of proteins expressed by cells that are either pro-apoptotic or anti-apoptotic, and normally the anti-apoptotic proteins inhibit activation of caspases, which are enzymes that chop proteins and DNA into little bits. The anti-apoptosis safety mechanism can be turned off internally, say when the cell is not receiving sufficient trophic signals. In this case, caspases are activated, proteins and DNA are fragmented, meltdown of cell structure and function ensues, and leftover cellular debris is rapidly cleared by phagocytosis.

It is estimated that during embryonic development of the nervous system, 50% or more of the neurons that are born die at a relatively young age, both before and after they have migrated to their ultimate destination and sent out axons to their targets. The sheer amount of apoptosis that goes on during early nervous system development is proof that it is a vital mechanism for weeding out noncompetitive neurons. To the extent that neurogenesis is a widespread phenomenon during adolescent brain development, we presume that apoptosis serves a similar weeding-out process for neurons that are born during adolescence. However, because the study of adolescent neurogenesis is relatively new, we really don't know how prominently apoptosis figures in the overall remodeling of the adolescent brain.

Apoptosis has a special and more subtle role in the creation of sexual dimorphisms in the developing nervous system (Forger, 2006). For cell groups like the rat AVPV and spinal nucleus of the bulbocavernosus (SNB), in which females have greater and fewer numbers of neurons than males, respectively, similar numbers of neurons are initially created during early development, and the sex differences in neuron number arise from differential rates of apoptosis. That is, females and males start out with equal numbers of neurons in the AVPV and SNB, but more AVPV cells die in males than in females, and conversely, more SNB cells die in females than in males (Forger, 2006). The AVPV and SNB dimorphisms are set up during prenatal and early postnatal development, and the differential amounts of cell death in these cell groups are under the control of testosterone, which is transiently elevated during the perinatal period in male rodents (Corbier, Kerdelhue, Picon, & Roffi, 1978). Testosterone accomplishes its death and survival mission in each cell group by regulating the expression of pro- and anti-apoptotic proteins, respectively (Forger, 2006).

How do these perinatal stories of sexual differentiation inform us about adolescent brain remodeling? Well, at least two sexual dimorphisms in the rat brain don't show up until adolescence. These sex differences are in the visual and medial prefrontal cortices, and in both cases, there are more neurons in adult males than in adult females. If you look at prepubertal rats, though, there are similar numbers of neurons in both regions in males and females. What happens during adolescence is that females lose cells in both the visual and prefrontal cortices, while the number of neurons in males remains stable (Markham, Morris, & Juraska, 2007; Nunez, Lauschke, & Juraska, 2001). By inference, then, apoptosis is the mechanism by which sexual dimorphisms in cortex arise during adolescence. Notably, if female rats are ovariectomized prepubertally, then the adolescent loss of neurons in the visual and prefrontal cortices does not occur (Koss, Lloyd, Sadowski, Wise, & Juraska, 2015; Nunez, Sodhi, & Juraska, 2002). Not only does this finding point to gonadal hormones as the driving force behind creation of sexual dimorphisms, but it is also an interesting role reversal for ovarian and testicular hormones. Ovarian hormones are given little credit for establishment of sexual dimorphisms during perinatal nervous system development (more on this in Chapter 6), yet here they are in adolescence being responsible for modulating cell survival and death and the subsequent sex difference in neuron number in cortical areas.

Migration

It seems likely that all these newly born cells during adolescence are going to have to migrate to their final destination from proliferative zones that are some distance away. Moreover, the possibility that mature neurons, born during early nervous system development, might have to move into a new neighborhood during adolescence cannot be excluded (as previously noted in the discussion of the increase in LC neurons during puberty; Pinos et al., 2001). For now, however, hard experimental evidence for or against long-distance migration of recently hatched neurons during adolescence is currently lacking. Thus, at this point, all we can say is that cellular migration probably plays a role in remodeling the adolescent brain, but the exact contribution of this particular mechanism is unclear.

Axonal Outgrowth

When neurons are born, they must extend axons of some length or another to be functional. Although we know that new neurons are born during adolescence, we do not know whether these pubertally born neurons become interneurons or projection neurons. Interneurons seem the easier, more efficient, and possibly more effective way to go, because they are positioned for agile and local modulation in any direction, and they do not have to take the time to extend an axon and hope that the signposts are in the right place for it to find its way to its correct spot. In addition, if adolescent brain development were analogous to metamorphosis, then one would expect that the nervous system retains most of the same neurons during the adolescent transition to adult physiology and behavior, but these neurons would be put to a different use. This change of jobs could be mediated by a developmental program of change in gene expression within the cell, by changes in afferent input, by modulation of cell excitability, or any combination of these (and other) possibilities. That said, it is certainly not beyond the nervous system to go for broke and generate completely new projections during adolescent development, even though that might seem the harder way to do it.

It turns out that axonal sprouting of existing projections and subsequent increases in synaptic connections during adolescent development have been well characterized in certain forebrain circuits. One example is the projection from the basolateral amygdala (BLA) to the prefrontal cortex in rodents. In this case, studies using a combination of retrograde and anterograde tract tracing methods show that the density of axonal projections from BLA to prefrontal cortex increases over adolescence, apparently in the absence of the addition of new projection neurons (Cunningham, Bhattacharyya, & Benes, 2002; Verwer, Van Vulpen, & Van Uum, 1996). This increase in innervation is paralleled by an increase in synapses and suggest a gain in excitatory or inhibitory input to the prefrontal cortex. Another well-studied example is the dramatic increase in dopaminergic input to the rat medial prefrontal cortex during adolescence (Benes, Taylor, & Cunningham, 2000). Here, the proportion of GABAergic neurons that is contacted by dopaminergic nerve terminals more than doubles throughout neonatal life and early adolescent development, accompanied by a late increase in the number of dopaminergic contacts on GABAergic neurons during late adolescence (Benes, Vincent, Molloy, & Khan, 1996). At the same time, the GABAergic cells themselves undergo a morphological transformation, acquiring additional dendritic branches (Vincent, Pabreza, & Benes, 1995). Dopaminergic influences on prefrontal GABAergic neurons are generally excitatory (Penit-Soria, Audinat, & Crepel, 1987), and so it appears that one mechanism by which the prefrontal cortex gains control of behavioral inhibition during adolescence is through an enhancement of excitatory inputs to inhibitory neurons.

Along these lines, an interesting observation was made with mice lacking both copies of the gene encoding a receptor for a molecule called netrin. Netrin is a signal that helps axonal growth cones navigate through their environment as they form synaptic connections. Mice with a genetic deficit that lack the receptor for netrin show decreased dendritic branching and connectivity of cells in the medial prefrontal cortex that often receive dopaminergic inputs (Grant et al., 2007). The interesting part to this story, however, is that these effects of the reduced receptor expression on neural structure in the prefrontal cortex are seen only after puberty (Manitt et al., 2011) and result in different levels of dopaminergic inputs to the adult prefrontal cortex (Hoops & Flores, 2017). Thus, together these data suggest proper axonal guidance is necessary for the shaping of forebrain circuits and their inputs during puberty and adolescence.

Synapse Proliferation and Synaptic Pruning

Concurrent with axonal outgrowth is synaptogenesis, as neurons are unlikely to go through the trouble of extending an axon without trying to establish synaptic connections with the target cell. This addition of synapses is sometimes accompanied by the subtraction of synapses, with synapse proliferation and pruning the yin-and-yang of changes in neuronal structural connectivity. More synaptic connections are initially made than eventually persist, and there is indisputable evidence that this pruning process occurs during adolescent brain development. In fact, synaptic pruning during the adolescent period was first described in the 1970s and 1980s (Huttenlocher, 1979) and was based on examination and quantification of human post-mortem tissue at the electron microscopic level, which is the gold standard for documenting synaptic connections between neurons. Yet, this aspect of adolescent brain development did not come to prominence until the more flashy structural magnetic resonance imaging (MRI) studies of the human adolescent brain were published in the 1990s (see Chapter 4 for the full story on this topic), even though one can only infer from MRI images that synaptic pruning underlies a decrease in gray matter volume. Both the electron microscopic and MRI data indicate that synaptic pruning during adolescence is a fairly widespread phenomenon, occurring in all six layers of cortex (Huttenlocher & Dabholkar, 1997) and virtually all cortical areas (Gogtay et al., 2004; Figure 3.2). Both methods also corroborate that the timing of synapse proliferation and elimination differs across cortical areas, with sensory and motor areas reaching adult-like levels earlier than associative and executive areas (Gogtay et al., 2004).

Between the electron microscopic and neural imaging levels of analysis is the circuit level of analysis, and this approach too has documented a curvilinear developmental pattern of synapse proliferation and pruning across adolescent development. Let us consider, as a specific example, the reciprocal connections between the BLA and medial prefrontal cortex (mPFC). As mentioned earlier in the axonal outgrowth section, tract-tracing studies in rats indicate that innervation of the mPFC from the BLA increases during the late preweaning/early adolescent period in rodents and is paralleled by an increase in synapses in the mPFC (Cunningham et al., 2002). A different group of researchers also employed methods to delineate structural connections in the rat brain and showed that innervation of the BLA from the mPFC decreases during later adolescence (Cressman et al., 2010). The authors of this study reasoned that some of these mPFC-to-BLA projecting neurons retract axons during late adolescence, leading to a corresponding reduction in synapses onto BLA neurons. So, here, we have an interesting case in which synapse proliferation and elimination are both spatially and temporally out of sync. Synapse proliferation occurs during early adolescence in the mPFC as a result of increased afferent input from the BLA, and then, perhaps paradoxically, the mPFC neurons that provide afferent input to the BLA retract some of their axons, resulting in a late adolescent reduction in synapses in

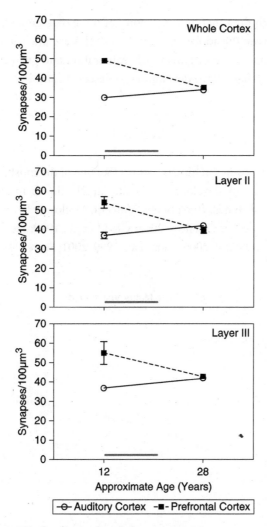

Figure 3.2. Synaptic density in the adolescent cortex.
Mean synaptic density (synapses/100 μm^3) in the human auditory (open circles) and prefrontal (closed squares) cortices (top panel) and specifically within cortical layer II (middle panel) and layer III (bottom panel) at approximately 12 and 28 years of age. Gray bar on the X-axis in each panel represents the approximate age span of adolescence. Redrawn from P. R. Huttenlocher & A. S. Dabholkar, 1997, Regional differences in synaptogenesis in human cerebral cortex, *Journal of Comparative Neurology, 387,* 167–178.

BLA. Although the functional outcomes of these divergent changes in connectivity between the adolescent mPFC and BLA are unclear, it shows these related and opposing mechanisms of proliferation and pruning play fundamental roles in shaping the developing adolescent brain.

Myelination

Structural MRI studies in humans reveal that one of the most robust features of adolescent brain development is the largely linear increase in white matter volumes (Benes, 1989; Benes, Vincent, Molloy, & Khan, 1994; Casey, Tottenham, Liston, & Durston, 2005; Giedd et al., 1999; Herting & Sowell, 2017; Lenroot & Giedd, 2006; Paus et al., 1999, 2001; Sowell, Trauner, Gamst,

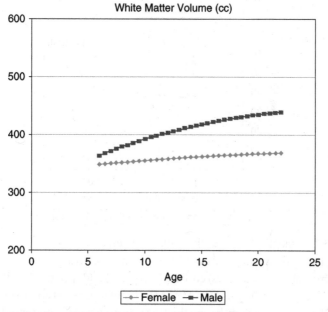

Figure 3.3. Increased myelination during adolescence.
Change in the overall volume (cc) of white matter in the human brain. Note the linear increase in myelination from childhood to adolescence and young adulthood. Reprinted from R. Lenroot & J. N. Giedd, 2006, Brain development in children and adolescents: Insights from anatomical magnetic resonance imaging, *Neuroscience and Biobehavioral Reviews, 30*, 718–729. Used with permission from Elsevier.

& Jernigan, 2002; Figure 3.3). Although the increase in white matter could be a reflection of increased axon myelination and/or axon caliber, either of these outcomes would contribute to greater conduction speeds of action potentials. Thus, these increases in white matter are usually considered an index of overall greater efficiency of neural transmission during adolescence.

Another consistent finding across studies is that the rate of change and overall white matter volume is greater in boys than in girls (De Bellis et al., 2001; Giedd et al., 1999; Herting et al., 2017; Lenroot & Giedd, 2010), begging the question if gonadal hormones are involved in these structural changes. In boys, the increase in white matter volume has been linked to testosterone and androgen receptor (AR) activity (Perrin et al., 2008). In this study, white matter volume was measured in adolescent males, some of whom carried a variation in their gene for AR marked by a higher number of CAG repeats (i.e., numerous repeats of the cytosine, adenine, and guanine DNA nucleotides within this gene), which is known to decrease AR transcriptional activity in the presence of testosterone. This study found a stronger positive correlation between testosterone levels and white matter volume in boys with the more efficient form of AR. Thus, the interaction of adolescent development, individual variation in androgen receptor function, and/or circulating hormonal levels may ultimately contribute to individual differences in nerve impulse conduction. Not only do these data indicate that changes in myelination contribute to adolescent brain remodeling but that, similar to some of the other previously discussed mechanisms, one factor driving these changes is the increase in gonadal hormone secretion at the onset of puberty.

Conclusion: The Renovated Home and Manicured Garden

We have seen how the same tools that were used to construct the nervous system during early development are pulled out again to remodel the brain during adolescent maturation. So, no new tricks, but it took us awhile to appreciate the extent to which the entire gamut of developmental mechanisms are called back into use to complete the remodeling required for the transition from childhood to adulthood. And it is worth noting again how long this takes: These processes of synapse proliferation, synaptic pruning, and myelination extend until well into the third decade of human life. Thus, just like home remodeling updates invariably take way longer than the contractor promised us it would, the adult brain takes longer to come to fruition than neuroscientists of 30 years ago ever imagined.

Recommended Reading

Giedd, J. N., & Rapoport, J. L. (2010). Structural MRI of pediatric brain development: What have we learned and where are we going? *Neuron, 67,* 728–734.

Khundrakpam, B. S., Lewis, J. D., Zhao, L., Chouinard-Decorte, F., & Evans, A. C. (2016). Brain connectivity in normally developing children and adolescents. *NeuroImage, 134,* 192–203.

Sanes D. H., Reh T. A., & Harris W. A. (2006). *Development of the nervous system* (2nd ed.). Burlington, MA: Elsevier Academic Press.

4

Remodeling the Adolescent Brain

From Local to Global

As the microscopic remodeling and pruning projects discussed in the last chapter transpire, the macroscopic contours of the adolescent brain begin to morph into their adult dimensions. When they first appeared in the scientific literature, these more global structural changes in the adolescent brain frankly surprised many neuroscientists. Their astonishment was not that the adolescent brain changed. After all, in the mid-20th century, the renowned Swiss developmental psychologist Jean Piaget had already recognized the qualitative leap in cognitive function that occurs in adolescence, when individuals become capable of abstract and hypothetical reasoning and logical thought. Instead, the shocking aspects of the early findings were twofold. First was the realization of the *extent* to which the adolescent brain is remodeled, and second was how *protracted* the process was, spanning well over a decade of human life. Given these rather significant findings, this leads to the obvious and slightly embarrassing question: How didn't we know this?

Magnetic Resonance Imaging

Our appreciation of these facets of adolescent brain development was made possible in part by magnetic resonance imaging (MRI). For a long time, the ability to study normative adolescent brain development in humans was limited by the lack of suitable technology. No one was eager to subject healthy children unnecessarily to the radiation and isotopes required in obtaining computerized tomography (CAT) or positron emission tomography (PET) scans, so imaging the brain at different ages throughout childhood and adolescence was not practical using these earlier methods. With the advent of MRI in the 1980s, which uses relatively harmless magnets and radio waves to create pictures of the brain with significant visual contrast between gray and white matter (Figure 4.1), there was finally a noninvasive, low-risk method of

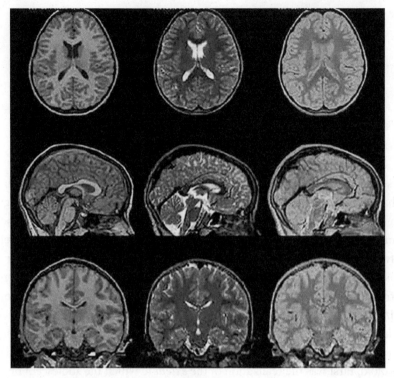

Figure 4.1. Magnetic resonance imaging (MRI).
Sample MRI brain scans from the MRI Study of Normal Brain Development.
Horizontal (top row), sagittal (middle row), and coronal (bottom row) scans
were captured using T1-weighted (left column), T2-weighted (middle column),
and proton density (PD) weighted (right column) acquisition protocols. Scans
like these are used to gather structural data regarding adolescent changes in
the volume of cortical and subcortical gray and white matter. More specifically,
in a T1-weighted image, there is a high contrast between brain areas with a
high fat content, such as white matter (appearing bright), and fluid-filled areas,
such as the ventricles (appearing dark). In a T2-weighted image, there is also
a high contrast between the white matter and the fluid-filled ventricles, but in
these images, the contrast is reversed, with the white matter appearing dark
and ventricles appearing bright. PD-weighted images provide good contrast
between gray and white matter, with gray matter and the ventricles appearing
relatively lighter than the white matter. Reprinted from A. C. Evans & the Brain
Development Cooperative Group, 2006, The NIH MRI study of normal brain
development, *NeuroImage, 30,* 184–202. Used with permission from Elsevier.

imaging the brain. Furthermore, given its comparative unobtrusive nature, the same individual could be reimaged repeatedly, permitting the production of valuable longitudinal data sets. This was a significant advancement, because cross-sectional data sets, which compare groups of *different* individuals at *different* ages, potentially suffer from large within-group variation, due to individual discrepancies in the timing of puberty, for instance. Thus, longitudinal studies more readily detect patterns of developmental change than cross-sectional studies (although regrettably longitudinal studies are still relatively rare in the neuroimaging field).

Over the past 25 years, structural MRI has permitted a clearer picture of where, when, and in what direction gross features of the brain, such as the volume of gray matter (i.e., cell bodies and synapses) and white matter (i.e., myelinated tracts and fibers), change over the course of adolescent development. In fact, a large multicenter project, the National Institutes of Health (NIH) MRI Study of Normal Brain Development, has been underway since 2006 (see Figure 4.1), with the objective of compiling a database of neurological, behavioral, and clinical variables over puberty and adolescence and to correlate features of brain maturation with behavioral milestones (Evans & the Brain Development Cooperative Group, 2006). As we shall see, this project (along with many other productive research groups) has begun to deliver on this objective.

What Have We Learned From MRI and Adolescent Brain Imaging?

At least three fundamental principles of adolescent brain development have already emerged from the MRI studies published since the late 1990s (Blakemore, 2012; Giedd & Rapoport, 2010; Giedd et al., 2015; Ladouceur, Peper, Crone, & Dahl, 2012). First, as previously mentioned, adolescent brain maturation is a protracted process, taking well over 10 years to complete (and in some cases extending into the third decade of life). As with any remodeling project, some systems are completed earlier than others are: the primary sensory and motor cortices mature first, followed by association and executive areas in frontal and temporal lobes. Thus, phylogenetically "older" brain areas mature earlier than "younger" areas (see Chapter 5 for a discussion of the functional implications of these temporal dissociations in the development of different parts of the brain). Second, the pattern of adolescent change in cortical gray matter volume is usually curvilinear, with an increase in volume occurring during late childhood and early adolescence, followed by a decrease in gray matter volume that occurs later in adolescence. As discussed in Chapter 3, these volumetric changes in gray matter might reflect an initial period of synaptic proliferation and a subsequent period of synapse elimination and pruning—consistent with the classic developmental studies using electron microscopy to quantify synaptic changes in postmortem human brain tissue (Huttenlocher & Dabholkar, 1997). Third, white matter volume increases linearly over adolescent development, likely resulting in a faster propagation of electrical signaling and, therefore, processing speed. Thus, taken together, the general picture that emerges from these fundamentals principles is that the nervous system that comes out at the other end of adolescent development is a more honed and efficient structure, potentially better set to meet the cognitive and emotional demands of young adulthood and beyond.

Cortical and Subcortical Structural Changes

From a bird's-eye perspective, total cerebral volume reaches its zenith at about 11 and 14 years of age in girls and boys, respectively (Lenroot & Giedd, 2006). Also, when all these structural changes are completed by young adulthood, males show an 8% to 10% greater overall cerebral volume than females, even after controlling for the sex differences in height and weight (Giedd, Snell et al., 1996). It is important to note, however, that this increase in total brain volume is not linear from infancy to adolescence. In fact, most of the gross maturation of the brain is completed by time we enter kindergarten, with about 95% of the total brain volume accomplished by 6 years of age (Dekaban & Sadowsky, 1978). As it turns out, however, that last 5% of brain development being wrapped up during adolescence is quite significant, particularly from a psychological functioning standpoint.

Looking at the cortex, or more specifically the thickness of the cortex, we see significant cortical *thinning* in the frontal and parietal cortices during adolescence. In both cortices, volumes peak about 11 years of age in girls and 12.5 years of age in boys, followed by a significant decline in thickness that tapers off in the 20s (Giedd et al., 1999; Figure 4.2). This thinning is not uniform across these cortices, however.

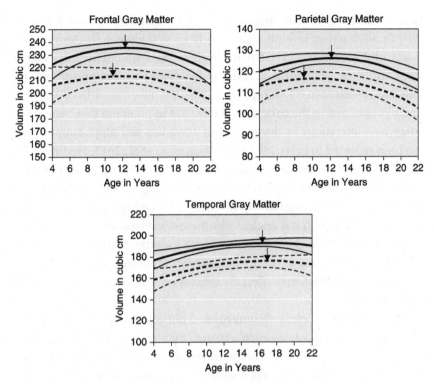

Figure 4.2. Adolescent-related cortical gray matter maturation. Adolescent-related changes in the gray matter volume of frontal, parietal, and temporal cortices in boys (solid lines) and girls (dotted lines). The arrows in each panel designate the peak volume obtained for that cortical region. These longitudinal data were collected from 145 scanned subjects in approximately 2-year intervals. Adapted and reprinted from R. Lenroot & J. N. Giedd, 2006, Brain development in children and adolescents: Insights from anatomical magnetic resonance imaging, Neuroscience and Biobehavioral Reviews, 30, 718–729. Used with permission from Elsevier.

For instance, dorsolateral prefrontal cortex is one of the latest areas to show this adolescent-related thinning pattern, while the dorsal parietal regions begin the earliest (Gogtay et al., 2004). The temporal cortex appears to be the late bloomer, in that peak volumes are obtained at about 16.5 years of age in both girls and boys, followed by less thinning than one sees in the frontal and parietal regions (Giedd et al., 1999; Figure 4.2).

The brain regions tucked under these cortices also demonstrate significant structural changes throughout adolescent development. Subcortical regions, such as the amygdala and hippocampus, show linear volumetric increases early in adolescence in both males and females (Figure 4.3). During mid- to late adolescence, however, females begin to show volumetric loss in these areas, while the volumetric increases in males tend to continue or level off into late adolescence (Goddings et al., 2014). Unlike the rather consistent findings obtained in the cortex, it is important to point out that these exact volumetric alterations in the adolescent amygdala and hippocampus have not been reported in every MRI study (Dennsion et al., 2013; Herting et al., 2014). One study found only volumetric increases in the right hippocampus and no changes in the amygdala (Dennsion et al., 2013), while another found growth in the right amygdala and no changes in the hippocampus (Herting et al., 2014). Although it is unclear why these discrepancies exist, these con- flicting data do highlight the ways in which experimental parameters used within each study, such as the age and number of subjects, and even the im- aging equipment itself, may affect the conclusions drawn from these types of neuroimaging studies.

The volumes of nucleus accumbens and dorsal striatum are also signifi- cantly altered during adolescence, although the structural changes seen here are opposite to those observed in the previously mentioned cortical and sub- cortical regions. Specifically, the nucleus accumbens, caudate, putamen, and globus pallidus largely show volumetric decreases, with slight differences in the steepness and shape of the curves in males and females (Goddings et al., 2014; Herting et al., 2014; Raznahan et al., 2014; Figure 4.3).

Interestingly, some of these volumetric changes in cortical and subcor- tical structures can be better predicted by the Tanner stage of the individual than by their chronological age (Goddings et al., 2014; Figure 4.3). As Tanner stage is a proxy for pubertal development, based on physical characteristics, such as testicular volume, breast growth, and the appearance of pubic hair (Marshall & Tanner, 1969, 1970), this would suggest these structural changes are in part influenced by pubertal changes in gonadal hormones (Peper, Hulshoff Pol, Crone, & van Honk, 2011). Indeed, recent studies have indi- cated that levels of testosterone and estradiol are better predictors of volume and rate of change in cortical thickness than even the Tanner stage (Herting et al., 2014, 2015). Data such as these suggest that gonadal hormones affect developmental trajectories of the adolescent brain and might help explain some of the sex differences observed in the maturation of these cortical and subcortical regions (Herting & Sowell, 2017; Wierenga et al., 2018). Not too surprisingly, however, the relationship between gonadal hormones and

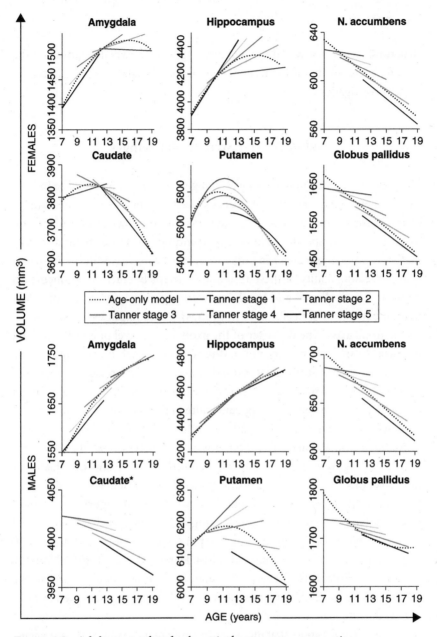

Figure 4.3. Adolescent-related subcortical gray matter maturation. Adolescent-related changes in the gray matter volumes of the amygdala, hippocampus, nucleus accumbens, caudate, putamen, and globus pallidus in females (top panels) and males (bottom panels). The dotted lines are the age-only models, while the different lines represent using the Tanner stage to model the structural changes within each subcortical region. Reprinted from A.-L. Goddings, K. L. Mills, L. S. Clasen, J. N. Giedd, R. M. Viner, & S.-J. Blakemore, 2014, The influence of puberty on subcortical brain development, *NeuroImage*, 88, 242–251. Used with permission from Elsevier.

structural changes in the adolescent brain appears to vary depending on the specific hormone in question, the sex of the individual, and the brain region under investigation.

White Matter Structural Changes

The previously noted morphological changes in gray matter would be indicative of changes in the number of neurons, the size of the neurons, the number of processes emanating from the neurons, or some combination thereof. Regardless of the specific cellular underpinnings for these changes in gray matter volume, these changes imply increases or decreases in the information processing ability of these functional groups of cortical or subcortical neurons. That's all well and good, but what about the movement of information between these cells and cell groups? Nerve impulses are sent along the neuron's axon. The diameter of the axon and its level of myelination are important variables in determining the speed at which nerve impulses are conducted, such that the greater the diameter and the greater the myelination (if any) of an axon, the greater the speed of the action potential traveling along that axon. In general, it appears white matter volumes increase during adolescence (Lebel & Beaulieu, 2011), with similar growth curves and trajectories in frontal, parietal, and temporal cortices (Giedd et al., 1999; Paus et al., 1999; Figure 4.4). Specific tracts, such as the corpus callosum, the major fiber tract that connects the right and left hemispheres of the brain, also show pubertal volumetric increases (Lenroot & Giedd, 2006; Figure 4.4). Similar to hormonal contributions to the shaping of gray matter changes, gonadal hormones have likewise been implicated in the pubertal-related increase in white matter volumes (Herting et al., 2014; Herting & Sowell, 2017; Menzies, Goddings, Whitaker, Blakemore, & Viner, 2015; Perrin et al., 2008), so the mechanisms contributing to these structural changes may be shared by both gray and white matter.

It is important to note that increases in white matter volume do not necessarily mean increased myelination surrounding each axon or axonal segment. That is, increases in axonal caliber could also result in measurable changes in white matter volumes without increased myelination per se (Perrin et al., 2008). Independent of the specific reason(s) for the increased white matter volume measured by MRI, be they based on actual myelin or axonal caliber, these increases suggest faster conduction speeds. Moreover, changes in white

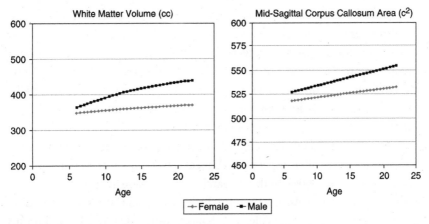

Figure 4.4. Adolescent-related white matter maturation.
Adolescent-related changes in cortical white matter volume (left panel) and mid-sagittal corpus callosum area (right panel) in males and females. Adapted and reprinted from R. Lenroot & J. N. Giedd, 2006, Brain development in children and adolescents: Insights from anatomical magnetic resonance imaging, *Neuroscience and Biobehavioral Reviews, 30*, 718–729. Used with permission from Elsevier.

matter volume and axonal caliber would have consequences for the synchrony of conduction, such that small changes in conduction speed between and within groups of neurons can lead to significant alterations in their oscillation frequencies and coupling of activity (Pajevic, Basser, & Fields, 2014). Taken together, developmental increases in white matter likely hasten and improve transmission between cell groups, helping keep our neural processing better coordinated and synchronous during adolescence.

Structure/Function Relationships

If we step back a bit and look at the structural data from a broader perspective, there are at least two important implications about function that can be drawn from these neuroanatomical studies. First, *bigger does not always mean better*. This point becomes self-evident when we consider the importance of cell death and synaptic pruning in the maturation of brain and behavior and the widespread loss of gray matter over the course of human adolescence, presumably leading to enhanced cognitive abilities. Second, *the journey may be as important as the destination.* Specifically, the dynamic pattern of gradual change in cortical gray and white matter volumes during childhood and adolescence suggests the timing of these volumetric changes are important. In support of this second assertion, converging lines of evidence from community and clinical samples indicate that the absolute thickness of cortex across development is not so much the important variable, but rather it is the *timing* and *rate* of cortical thickening and thinning that are the clues to individual differences in outcome. For instance, a fascinating study linked these two aspects of cortical development to general intelligence (Shaw et al., 2006). In this research, subjects were imaged repeatedly at roughly 2-year intervals, and their intelligence quotient (IQ) was assessed by the Wechsler Intelligence Scale. The subjects were categorized based on IQ range as having superior (121–149), high (109–120), or average (83–108) intelligence. The trajectories of cortical thickness were clearly different among these groups. To their surprise, the researchers found that the subjects with superior intelligence actually started out with a thinner prefrontal cortex at age 7, but by the time they were in their early teens, ended up with a thicker cortex in some prefrontal regions. And, the age at peak cortical thickness was different among the groups, with the peak occurring several years later in the subjects with superior intelligence. Then, when they analyzed the rate of cortical thickening and pruning, the subjects with superior intelligence showed steeper curves; that is, they showed both a more rapid thickening and a more rapid thinning of cortex over the course of adolescence (Shaw et al., 2006; Figure 4.5). It is fascinating to consider what this means. Perhaps "superior intellect" is associated with both the ability to generate more neurons/synapses early on, maximizing the potential for plasticity or options, and later on being more responsive to experiential factors to prune synapses without optimal inputs and stimulation.

Normal Versus Abnormal Development

The normative patterns of adolescent brain development that have been revealed by MRI studies over the past 25 years are already being compared to those of clinical populations to help understand the events that go awry in neurodevelopmental disorders associated with puberty and adolescence. A psychopathology commonly associated with adolescence is schizophrenia, which typically emerges during late adolescence or early adulthood (Lee,

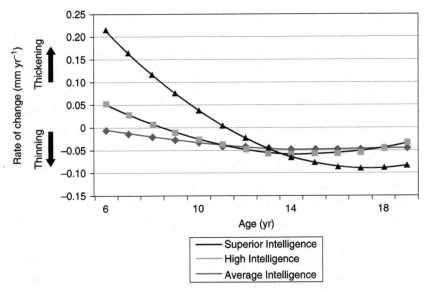

Figure 4.5. Cortical maturation and IQ.
These data show the rate of cortical change during adolescence and its association with superior, high, or average intelligence. Notably, those with superior intelligence showed both a faster thickening and thinning of the cortex during adolescent development than those with high or average intelligence. Reprinted from P. Shaw, D. Greenstein, J. Lerch, L. Clasen, R. Lenroot, N. Gogtay, . . . J. Giedd, 2006, Intellectual ability and cortical development in children and adolescents, *Nature, 440,* 676–679. Used with permission from Springer Nature.

Heimer et al., 2014). An elegant longitudinal neuroimaging study compared the dynamic pattern of cortical thinning in healthy adolescents to adolescents with childhood onset schizophrenia (COS). These subjects were scanned at 2½-year intervals between 13 and 18 years of age. The MRI scans revealed that the rate of cortical gray matter loss in the group affected with schizophrenia was about 4% per year, as compared to the 1% observed in the control group (Thompson et al., 2001; Vidal et al., 2006). More specifically, the parietal and medial frontal cortices appeared to be affected in the early stages of COS; namely, these cortical areas were already thinner in COS subjects than in controls at the first scan. Conversely, dorsolateral prefrontal, temporal, and cingulate cortices appeared to be affected later in COS, with differences in cortical thickness between COS and unaffected subjects not seen until the later scans. Since absolute cortical thickness in these areas was less in COS subjects than controls, it's unclear whether it's the rate of cortical thinning that is the relevant variable underlying functional differences between the groups (as in the Shaw et al., 2006, study in the context of IQ), or whether it's how thin that cortex actually is. Future studies will hopefully reveal the answer.

One historical note, about 35 years ago, before all these MRI studies, Irwin Feinberg proposed that a defect in the normal process of synaptic pruning was responsible for the emergence of schizophrenia in late adolescence (Feinberg, 1982). His hypothesis was based in part on the work of Huttenlocher and his electron microscopic studies of post mortem human brains showing the synaptic pruning in the cortex during adolescence (Huttenlocher, 1979). Feinberg couldn't state explicitly whether too little or too much pruning was the problem with schizophrenia, or whether pruning too early or too late was the culprit, but his hypothesis was well ahead of its time, and his thinking apparently spot on about the potential significance of this developmental process in the etiology of schizophrenia.

In contrast to COS, autism spectrum disorder (ASD) is associated with a *leftward* shift in the timing of the increase in cortical thickness and subsequent thinning (Wallace, Dankner, Kenworthy, Giedd, & Martin, 2010; Figure 4.6). In particular, the degree of cortical thinning is greater in the left temporal and parietal cortices, at least in high functioning individuals with ASD compared to typically developing adolescents (Wallace et al., 2010). Because ASD appears well before puberty and adolescence, the advancement of the inverted-U pattern of changes in cortical thickness and the more robust thinning seen with autism are likely to be part of a more global aberration in neural development that is set in motion from a very early age. Regardless, these kinds of datasets illustrate how a greater appreciation of typical, normative adolescent brain development can provide a valuable framework for better understanding the structural markers, or even mediators, of various devastating development disorders and psychological dysfunctions.

Some Limitations of MRI Data

It is undeniable that structural MRI, and related neuroimaging technologies, have allowed neuroscientists and psychologists to expose the enormous amount of development exhibited by the adolescent nervous system.

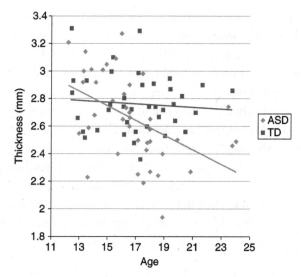

Figure 4.6. Cortical maturation and autism spectrum disorder (ASD). A study reporting increased cortical thinning in the temporal/fusiform gyrus in adolescents with ASD (lighter gray line and data points) compared to typically developing (TD) adolescents (darker gray line and data points). Reprinted from G. L. Wallace, N. Dankner, L. Kenworthy, J. N. Giedd, & A. Martin, 2010, Age-related temporal and parietal cortical thinning in autism spectrum disorders, *Brain, 133,* 3746–3754. Used with permission from Oxford University Press.

However, there are some limitations as to what these studies can tell us about morphological brain maturation.

One limitation is the resolution. Although resolution in neuroimaging continues to increase with the development of more powerful scanners, one has to remember that a large number of cells make up each one of those voxels in a brain scan. In other words, although a picture might be worth a thousand words, a voxel is likely more than a thousand cells. This means that the cellular bases of these gross structural changes based on MRI scans are largely unknown. It will be interesting to see whether running similar imaging studies in nonhuman animal models will allow us to understand more fully what MRI scans mean at a cellular level by combining MRI studies with meticulous histological studies on the same tissue.

Another limitation of structural MRI data is the difficulty in ascribing functional changes and outcomes to the thickening and thinning of brain tissue. Obviously, *functional* MRI (fMRI) can help us appreciate these structure/function issues, but it's hard sometimes not to just interpret structural MRI data with a neo-phrenology mindset, thinking that the bigger spot of gray matter in cortical region "X" is equal to a bigger change in function mediated by that portion of cortical region "X." Indeed, as the cortical thinning data are revealing to us, less may mean more, and the pruning of cells and synapses may actually make a circuit more streamlined and proficient.

Finally, good MRI images are dependent on immobile subjects—not a trivial problem when dealing with children and young adolescent individuals, not to mention children with neuropsychological disorders. Although improvements in scanning technology and constantly improving algorithms and statistical models are helping to reduce the movement artifacts inherent in MRI data collection, these seemingly small issues can turn into big issues when comparing scans across ages as well as across studies.

Neuroimaging and Adolescent Brain Maturation: We Have Only Just Begun

In this chapter, we focused on a single neuroimaging technique suitable to structural analyses. It is important to remember, however, that other imaging methodologies, such as diffusion tensor imaging and fMRI, continue to provide valuable information regarding the connectivity and functional relationships that emerge from these structural changes, revealing how the adolescent brain operates differently than at other stages of life. Furthermore, the MRI technique itself still has quite a bit to teach us from the scans already analyzed and archived. Researchers are reanalyzing previous MRI data sets to assess structural covariance between brain areas within an individual (Alexander-Bloch, Giedd, & Bullmore, 2013). These analyses attempt to quantify how brain regions might be maturing in tandem and whether these contemporaneous changes have functional implications for the development of specific sensory or cognitive abilities within an individual. For example, in the visual pathway, the sizes of the optic tract, lateral geniculate, and visual cortex are positively correlated within a person, suggesting that a structural relationship among brain areas indicates connectedness (Andrews, Halpern, & Purves, 1997). As proof-in-principle in a developing population, a similar phenomenon was noted in language areas, with anterior and posterior cortical regions in the left hemisphere showing covariance in size as children mature (Lerch et al., 2006). In the context of adolescent development, this type of analysis showed the fronto-temporal areas exhibit "maturational coupling," such that the rate of change was more similar in frontal and temporal regions than in sensorimotor cortices, and that this coupling was between areas that had structural connections (Raznahan et al., 2011). Thus, instead of looking at regions in isolation, these newer analyses are investigating potential synchrony of maturation across regions and, importantly, what this synchrony (or asynchrony) in maturational coupling may mean to the developing adolescent brain (Sotiras et al., 2017).

The field has come a long way since the late 1990s when the first MRI-based longitudinal reports of structural changes in the adolescent brain were published (Giedd et al., 1999; Paus et al., 1999; Sowell et al., 1999). Although more surprises definitely await, many surprises have already been revealed, such as cortical thinning as a hallmark of adolescent brain maturation. As technical innovations continue to improve scanner capabilities and more sophisticated computational models are brought to bear on imaging data (Goldenberg & Galvan, 2015; Kundu et al., 2018), we will undoubtedly gain a greater insight into normal adolescent brain development and begin to appreciate how perturbations in these developmental processes lead to neuropsychological dysfunctions in adolescents and adults.

Recommended Reading

Foulkes, L., & Blakemore, S-J. (2018). Studying individual differences in human adolescent brain development. *Nature Neuroscience, 21*, 315–323.

Petersen, S. E., & Sporns, O. (2015). Brain networks and cognitive architectures. *Neuron, 88*, 207–219.

Somerville, L. H. (2016). Searching for signatures of brain maturity: What are we searching for? *Neuron, 92*, 1164–1167.

5

Executive Function

What Were You Thinking?

As adolescence progresses, with the ripples and waves of brain maturation occurring out of sight under the skull, a cluster of more conspicuous cognitive changes becomes apparent (Spear, 2010; Steinberg, 2010). For instance, teenagers acquire increased capacity for selective attention, goal-directed behavior, impulse inhibition, skill in reading and interpreting social cues, regulatory control of emotions, and abstract thought (Blakemore & Choudhury, 2006; Burnett, Sebastian, Kadosh, & Blakemore, 2011; Kilford, Garrett, & Blakemore, 2016; Luna, Garver, Urban, Lazar, & Sweeney, 2004; Murty, Calabro, & Luna, 2016; Sebastian, Burnett, & Blakemore, 2008; Sturman & Moghaddam, 2011). These cognitive abilities all fall under the general rubric of executive function or the capacity to control and coordinate thoughts and behavior. Executive functions are largely orchestrated within the frontal lobe, in particular by the most anterior third of the frontal lobe known as prefrontal cortex (Dalley, Cardinal, & Robbins, 2004; Goldman-Rakic, 1996). Although the prefrontal cortex often takes center stage in any discussion of cognitive maturation during adolescence, this brain region does not operate in isolation. There are numerous areas whose interactions with the prefrontal cortex are vitally important in these shifts in cognition, but here we will only focus on a couple, namely the amygdala and striatum.

As reviewed in Chapters 3 and 4, we are starting to get a solid understanding of the basic building blocks of neural development as well as the more global structural changes that happen in the adolescent brain. However, going from these basic structural elements to making inferences about why an adult may be better than a teenager at self-regulation and management of emotions remains a rather large leap, and it is going to take some time before this complete story reveals itself. Nevertheless, progress is being made, and as the plot thickens, we are starting to get a better understanding of the relationship between adolescent brain development and cognitive maturation.

One part of this story begins with the gruesome and captivating account of Phineas Gage. In a workplace accident in 1848, Mr. Gage's prefrontal cortex was damaged and disconnected from the rest of his brain by an iron tamping rod that penetrated the left side of his face and emerged out the right side of the top of his head (Damasio, Grabowski, Frank, Galaburda, & Damasio, 1994). Yes, you read that correctly. Amazingly, Mr. Gage recovered rather quickly from the physical injury, but psychologically, he was never the same. Formerly a mild-mannered and reliable worker, Mr. Gage became emotionally volatile, unfocused, irascible, irreverent, and disrespectful after his injury. His personality had changed, and his misfortune gave us valuable clues as to the crucial role the prefrontal cortex plays in normal cognitive and emotional function. Now, more than 150 years later, thanks in large part to case studies of people with prefrontal cortical lesions and functional MRI (fMRI) studies (Figure 5.1), we have a reasonably sophisticated understanding of prefrontal cortex function and, specifically, what types of cognitive tasks rely on this region.

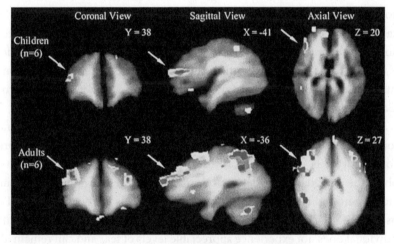

Figure 5.1. Functional magnetic resonance imaging (fMRI).
Sample fMRI brain scans in a coronal (left images), sagittal (middle images), and axial (right images) view from a study testing spatial working memory in children (top row of images) and adults (bottom row of images). Highlighted areas on the brain are those regions showing a change in activity during execution of the task. Reprinted from B. J. Casey, J. Giedd, & K. M. Thomas, 2000, Structural and functional brain development and its relation to cognitive development, *Biological Psychology, 54,* 241–257. Used with permission from Elsevier.

The prefrontal cortex can be roughly divided into three major regions: dorsolateral, orbitofrontal, and medial. The dorsolateral prefrontal cortex is associated with executive functions related to goal-directed behavior and planning for the future (Ridderinkhof, van den Wildenberg, Segalowitz, & Carter, 2004). Individuals with damage to this area have impaired judgment, focus, and pursuit of goals (Forbes & Grafman, 2010). The orbitofrontal prefrontal cortex mediates face perception and emotional intelligence (Hahn & Perrett, 2014), and when it malfunctions, the affected individual is moody, distractible, and doesn't read others' expressions, body language, and emotionality very well (Operskalski, Paul, Colom, Barbey, & Grafman, 2015). Finally, the medial prefrontal cortex (mPFC) is related to spontaneity, including spontaneous speech and prosody (Whitney et al., 2008). Individuals with damage to this region come across as apathetic (Huey et al., 2015). If we imagine the executive function deficits that would ensue from global malfunction of the prefrontal cortex, we would see someone who is impulsive, who has difficulty paying attention, who can't easily control their own emotions or accurately read those of others, and who falls short in thinking through the consequences of their own behavior. Hmm—sound like a teenager? It is becoming clearer that stereotypical teenage behavior is related to "immaturity" of the prefrontal cortex. However, there is more to the story than that, as it appears the interaction of the prefrontal cortex with other subcortical areas crucial for emotional function, such as the amygdala and striatum, also play a significant role (Casey, Getz, & Galvan, 2008).

As we have already introduced you to the prefrontal cortex and its function, now let us turn briefly to the amygdala and striatum. Just as the prefrontal cortex is synonymous with executive function, the quintessential job of the amygdala is to detect and process fearful and menacing stimuli and add emotional context to an experience (Phelps & LeDoux, 2005). For instance, if an individual has brain damage restricted to the amygdala, that individual does not experience appreciable levels of fear and can remain abnormally placid in the face of extremely fearful situations. Similar to the prefrontal cortex, the amygdala also is comprised of many subregions, including the central and basolateral nuclei (Phelps & LeDoux, 2005), each with their unique characteristics, connectivity, and functions. Finally, rounding out this triad, the striatum, particularly the bottom or ventral portion, is most popular for its role in processing information pertinent to motivation and reward (Ernst & Fudge, 2009). Perhaps not too surprisingly, this area figures large in the research of those studying addiction and drug abuse (which we will discuss in Chapter 8). With these introductions out of the way, let us describe the interaction among these regions and how their different developmental trajectories may give rise to a troubling aspect of adolescent behavior: risk-taking.

The Triadic Model and Risk-Taking

Although risk-taking may have a negative connotation—say, in the context of a teenager risking their life by getting a ride home from a party with an intoxicated friend—we may nevertheless owe the propagation of our species to the taking of risks. That is, imagine if you had to leave the comfort of your familiar, stable home environment and strike out on your own to find potential mates, especially when you are not yet fully mature. This would require a certain amount of moxie, and it would help if you happened to be a little less risk averse at such a time. Thus, seeing risk-taking through this lens, it appears that the increase in risky behaviors that many animals show during puberty may be normal behavioral changes ultimately driven by the grander purpose of reproductive success. Of course, just because something is natural does not mean it is safe, and that may be why a number of adolescents find themselves in serious, life-threatening situations. In other words, risk-taking can be risky, and hence its negative reputation may be well deserved.

So, what are the neural substrates that contribute to this shift in behavior and what makes the adolescent brain seem so perfectly tuned to make risky decisions? The answers to these questions appear to be, at a minimum, the prefrontal cortex, amygdala, and striatum and particularly their differential developmental trajectories, connections, and interactions.

A number of theories and hypotheses provide strong rationales for the substantial emotional and behavioral changes observed during adolescence (reviewed in Sturman & Moghaddam, 2011). Here, we will highlight just one of these models as an example, the triadic model and particularly its role in the context of risk-taking behavior (Ernst & Fudge, 2009; Ernst, Pine, & Hardin, 2006; Richards, Plate, & Ernst, 2012). At its core, the triadic model simply views motivated behaviors (i.e., behaviors in response to stimuli in an effort to reach a goal) as the interaction of two sets of opposing behaviors: *approach* and *avoidance* behaviors, with the third part of the triad, *modulation*, ultimately tipping the balance for an approach or avoidance behavior to be elicited. Although these three factors are separated conceptually, they overlap quite a bit practically. These three systems are mediated primarily by three separate neural substrates, which, as you may have guessed, are the striatum (approach), amygdala (avoidance), and prefrontal cortex (modulation). The balance between these systems allows measured decisions to be made, while an imbalance in these systems leads to a lopsided decision, perhaps one with a little too much approach and not enough avoidance (Figure 5.2). If the striatum, amygdala, and prefrontal cortex all matured in parallel and at the same rate with one another, then motivated behaviors would be "balanced" throughout one's development. The maturation of these neural nodes, however, is not in lockstep, and their differential maturational rates during adolescence may underlie the shifts in approach and avoidance behaviors.

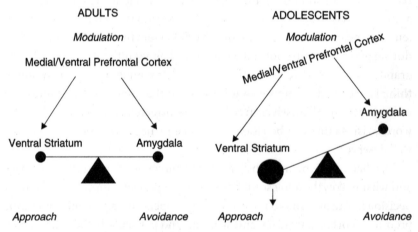

Figure 5.2. Triadic model. A model of why adolescent and adult motivated behaviors, such as risk taking, might be balanced differently.
During adulthood, approach (in part mediated by the ventral striatum), avoidance (in part mediated by the amygdala), and modulation (in part mediated by the prefrontal cortex) are in balance, while during adolescence, due to uneven maturation of these systems, more approach behaviors might result, particularly those behaviors associated with obtaining something with a high reward value. Reprinted from M. Ernst & J. L. Fudge, 2009, A developmental neurobiological model of motivated behavior: Anatomy, connectivity and ontogeny of the triadic nodes, *Neuroscience and Biobehavioral Reviews, 33,* 367–382. Used with permission from Elsevier.

The Metamorphosis of the Adolescent Brain Revisited

As alluded to in Chapter 4, structural imaging studies have revealed that subcortical areas generally finish maturing sooner than cortical areas (Giedd & Rapoport, 2010; Gogtay et al., 2004). In the striatum, for instance, most of the structural changes occur early in development and are fully mature by adolescence (Muftuler et al., 2011; Sowell, Thompson, Colin, Jernigan, & Toga, 1999). Similarly, in the amygdala, there is a slight increase in volume between childhood and adolescence, particularly on the left side of the brain (Giedd, Vaituzis et al., 1996; Payne, Machado, Bliwise, & Bachevalier, 2010; Tottenham & Sheridan, 2010). The prefrontal cortex, on the other hand, is one of the last cortical structures to reach full maturity, with estimates that gross structural maturation isn't complete until after the second decade of life (Giedd et al., 1999; Giedd & Rapoport, 2010; Shaw et al., 2008; see Figure 4.2). Thus, when you put all this structural imaging data together, the general picture that emerges is that an individual in the throes of adolescence has a relatively mature striatum and amygdala, and thus the approach and avoidance nodes are largely online, but the prefrontal node responsible for modulating or gating these approach and avoidance behaviors is still relatively immature.

Parallel with these morphing gray matter regions, white matter tracts, the parts of the nerve cells connecting the islands of gray matter together, also show adolescent-related maturation. Recall from Chapter 4 that these changes in the white matter fibers are usually more linear in nature, compared with the inverted-U kind observed with gray matter (Giedd et al., 1999; Lebel & Beaulieu, 2011; Paus et al., 1999; Schmithorst & Yuan, 2010; see Figure 4.4). As we mentioned before, it is not clear whether the growth of these tracts is due to increases in myelination and/or increases in the diameter of the axons (Paus, 2010), but either possibility would lead to a faster flow of nerve impulses and thus presumably greater speeds of communication between brain areas.

Along with these adolescent-related structural changes in gray and white matter, fMRI has begun to shed light on the differences in the activity of these areas during adolescent development. For example, adolescent individuals respond with greater neural activity in the striatal region following or anticipating a reward than adults (Ernst et al., 2005; Galvan, 2010; Galvan et al., 2006; Geier, Terwilliger, Teslovich, Velanova, & Luna, 2010), while adults show greater activation within the amygdala when a reward is withheld (Ernst et al., 2005). In essence, therefore, the adolescent striatum displays greater activity after a positive outcome and less amygdalar activation following a negative outcome compared to the adult striatum. In the context of the frontal cortex, adults show more focal activation following reward than adolescents, perhaps indicating a more efficient, honed response in the mature frontal cortex (Galvan et al., 2006).

Taken together, these studies of structural and functional changes suggest that in situations requiring an adolescent to evaluate information under risky circumstances, the approach and avoidance nodes are not being "filtered" or gated by the frontal cortex in the same way in the adolescent as they are in the adult. Although there are undoubtedly more elements needed to fully explain developmental shifts in risk-taking and impulsive behaviors, the triadic model does provide a framework to begin to understand and appreciate why teens may behave in more risky and impulsive ways than adults.

It is important to note that studies utilizing animal models have allowed scientists to begin to dig deeper into functional changes in the adolescent brain, particularly in regards to neurochemical alterations in areas like the prefrontal cortex and ventral striatum. Similar to the human studies, experiments on rodents have shown that adolescent rats perform more poorly on tests that assess executive function, such as attentional set shifting and reversal learning (Newman & McGaughy, 2011). In general, adolescent rats and mice also appear to be more impulsive than their more mature counterparts (Adriani & Laviola, 2003; Burton & Fletcher, 2012; Doremus-Fitzwater, Barreto, & Spear, 2012; Lukkes, Norman, Meda, & Andersen, 2016; Pinkston & Lamb, 2011). Accompanying these behavioral changes, concentrations of specific neurotransmitters ebb and flow in synapses within the adolescent and adult rat brain. Specifically, extracellular norepinephrine concentrations were found to be higher in the left mPFC of adolescent compared to adult rats, while the opposite difference was found in the right mPFC (Staiti et al., 2011). In the nucleus accumbens, dopamine transients (i.e., subsecond changes in dopamine concentration) are similar in adolescent and adult rats. However, after exposure to repeated, brief social interactions, dopamine transients in the adult accumbens decrease, while the transients in the adolescent show no such habituation (Robinson, Zitzman, Smith, & Spear, 2011). The exact correlation of these neurochemical fluctuations to changes in adolescent executive function, risk-taking, and impulsivity remains elusive, as well as what functional implications these changes may have for various models of cognitive change, including the triadic model. These data do indicate, however, that animal models could provide researchers with an opportunity to probe how adolescent-related changes observed in more "macro" neuroimaging studies may translate to the more "micro" neurochemical and biophysical profiles and properties of adolescent neurons and synapses.

Pubertal Hormones and Executive Maturation in Boys and Girls

From the many previously discussed experimental studies, it is clear that adolescence represents a period of life marked by changes in many aspects of executive functioning (Blakemore & Choudhury, 2006; Yurgelun-Todd, 2007). These changes are not necessarily linked to chronological age nor are the rates of change similar in boys and girls. A more direct regulator of these alterations may be the massive pubertal-related rise in gonadal hormone levels associated with puberty (Berenbaum & Beltz, 2011; Romeo, 2003; Sisk & Zehr, 2005). As discussed in other chapters, the increases in gonadal hormones, such as testosterone and estradiol, can affect brain development in both transient and permanent ways (see Chapters 3, 4, and 6). The role that these hormonal changes may play in driving the adolescent structural and functional modifications, within and between the sexes, is gaining wider attention (Blakemore, Burnett, & Dahl, 2010; Herting & Sowell, 2017; Lenroot & Giedd, 2010). For instance, total gray matter volumes are negatively correlated with estradiol in girls, while the opposite correlation is noted with testosterone in boys (Peper et al., 2009). Moreover, the higher the estradiol level in periadolescent girls (10–15 years of age), the greater the decreases in prefrontal volume, but the greater the increases in medial frontal areas (Peper et al., 2009). Although these anatomical data highlight the importance of appreciating the far-reaching, and sometimes diametrically opposed, influences of gonadal hormones on brain structure, the impact of these hormones on neuronal *function* are less understood. One study, however, has drawn attention to just how complex this interaction of sex, hormones, and age can be and what this interaction may mean for emotionality (Goddings, Heyes, Bird, Viner, & Blakemore, 2012). In this experiment, adolescent girls (11–14 years of age) were given scenarios to read that tapped into either social emotions (embarrassment and guilt) or basic emotions (disgust and fear), and their neural responses were measured using fMRI. The pubertal stage of these girls was also evaluated by various means, including a measurement of their hormone concentrations. Not surprisingly, brain regions known to be important in processing social emotions, such as the prefrontal cortex, were activated to a greater extent by the social versus basic emotion scenarios. Interestingly, however, the activity in these areas was highest in the girls with the highest hormone levels, independent of age (Goddings et al., 2012). These data hint at the rich complexity of factors that shape some aspects of emotionality during adolescence and the need to approach both structural and functional studies of adolescent brain development with a sensitivity to age, sex, and hormonal variables.

Under Pressure

Along with these "internal factors" that modulate executive function, there are many "external factors," such as stress, that have been shown to tweak our likelihood of making poor or risky decisions. Studies in adults, for instance, have reported that risky decision-making increases significantly under conditions of high stress (Lighthall, Mather, & Gorlick, 2009; Phuong & Galvan, 2017; Porcelli & Delgado, 2009; van den Bos, Harteveld, & Stoop, 2009). In fact, at least in men, the more stress reactive one is, the riskier one's decisions may become under stressful circumstances (van den Bos et al., 2009). A study in teenage boys and girls has expanded on this topic, showing that a greater incidence of risky decisions is made in adolescents who self-report high levels of stress compared to those who report low levels (Galvan & McGlennen, 2012). This effect of stress was not seen in these teens when they were completing a response inhibition task, suggesting some specificity of the domain of executive function that is affected by stress in adolescents (Galvan & McGlennen, 2012). Although the neural bases of these stress effects on decision-making are somewhat murky, neuroimaging data in adults hint at a role for the striatum and frontal cortex (Porcelli, Lewis, & Delgado, 2012). It will be interesting to see what similarities or differences will be noticed when these types of imaging experiments are done on stressed out teenagers.

Under Peer Pressure

Another layer of complexity that must be taken into consideration when discussing adolescent risk-taking and impulsivity is the context in which it frequently occurs, namely the social context. The importance of peers on risk-taking by adolescents was underscored in an elegant study by Gardner and Steinberg (2005). In their study, a set of questionnaires and behavioral tasks was administered to individuals in three age groups: adolescents (13–16 years of age), youths (18–22 years of age), and adults (24 years of age and older). Importantly, these assessments were taken when the subjects were either alone or with friends. The questionnaires assessed risk preference and risky decision-making, while the behavioral test measured risk-taking by having subjects play a video game, called Chicken, which had them decide when to stop a car as a traffic light turned from green to yellow. It was found that young individuals were more "risky" than adults as indexed by both the risky decision-making questionnaire and their performance on the Chicken video game, indicating that risk-taking generally decreases with age (Gardner & Steinberg, 2005; Figure 5.3). However, the neat part of this study was how these individuals did on these measures when tested in the presence of friends. Under these conditions, everybody showed more riskiness than when tested alone, but this increase in peer-induced risk-taking was at its maximum among the adolescent subjects (Gardner & Steinberg, 2005; Figure 5.3). These data indicate that the only person riskier than an adolescent is an adolescent in the presence of friends.

This same research group also examined brain activity via fMRI in adolescents (14–18 years of age), young adults (19–22 years of age), and adults (24–29 years of age) while participating in a driving simulation game similar to the previously mentioned Chicken. Again, these subjects "drove" in the presence or absence of a couple of friends. Similar to the previously described study, adolescents displayed the highest level of risk-taking when tested in the presence of their friends (Chein, Albert, O'Brien, Uckert, & Steinberg, 2011). Moreover, reward-related brain circuitry, like the ventral striatum, showed higher levels of activation in the adolescent subjects under peer conditions than the other older age groups. On the other hand, adults (either with or without peers present) showed

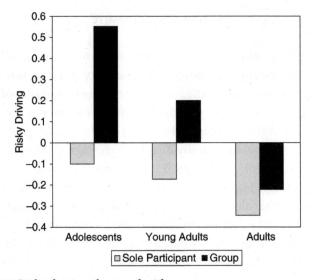

Figure 5.3. Risky driving alone and with peers.
Risky driving scores (higher scores indicate higher risk-taking) in adolescents
(13–16 years old), youths (18–22 years old), and adults (24 years old and
older) tested in a game of "Chicken" either alone (sole participant; grey
bars) or with two same-age group peers (group; black bars). Reprinted
from M. Gardner & L. Steinberg, 2005, Peer influence on risk taking, risk
preference, and risky decision making in adolescence and adulthood: An
experimental study, *Developmental Psychology, 41,* 625–635. Used with
permission from American Psychological Association.

greater neural activation in areas associated with cognitive control, such
as the prefrontal cortex (Chein et al., 2011). These results suggest that
increased risk-taking, at least in mid- and late-adolescent individuals,
might be mediated in part by adolescents finding risk-taking more rewarding while in the presence of their friends (Chein et al., 2011). One
caveat when discussing these functional imaging data is the age of the
"adolescent" subjects. Pfeifer et al. (2011) found children entering adolescence (13 years of age) show greater activity in the ventral striatum correlated with less susceptibility to peer influence in the context of risk-taking.
Hence, as with any research, the devil is in the details, and these details
can be important in the interpretation of the data. However, it would generally appear that differential activation of these brain regions might play
a role in adolescent changes in risk-taking.

Roper v. Simmons

The previously highlighted normative adolescent-related changes in risk-taking and impulsivity have led to many debates and controversies in the context of public policy making and practice, particularly in the juvenile justice system (Cauffman & Steinberg, 2000; Steinberg, 2003, 2009a, 2009b). One hot-button issue is whether adolescent individuals should be held responsible for their actions when their impulse control coordination may be a bit clumsy. The button has only grown hotter when these questions are posed in conjunction with the recent discoveries from developmental neuroscience showing the continued maturation of prefrontal and other cortical regions during adolescence and their relationship to impulsivity (Giedd, 2008; Shannon et al., 2011; Steinberg, 2009b).

A classic example of this debate swirling around these issues of adolescent criminal culpability was a groundbreaking case argued at the U.S. Supreme Court in 2004. Briefly, Christopher Simmons, a 17-year-old high school junior, had committed murder, was tried (after his 18th birthday), and sentenced to death. Although it was clear that he committed the crime, the case questioned the constitutionality of capital punishment for those individuals who committed their crime prior to turning 18 years of age. The defense argued he was "very impulsive" and "susceptible to being manipulated": in essence, an adolescent (*Roper v. Simmons*, 2005). The American Psychological Association (APA), the largest professional organization representing psychologists in the United States, weighed in on the case by sending briefs to the Supreme Court emphasizing the research on adolescent risk-taking and its relation to continued brain maturation (APA, 2004). For example, Arguments A2 and A3 in the APA brief were "adolescent decision-makers on average are less future-oriented and less likely to consider properly the consequences of their actions" and "neuropsychological research demonstrates that the adolescent brain has not reached adult maturity," respectively (APA, 2004). Although it is unclear whether APA's input affected the outcome of this case, the Supreme Court did countermand the death penalty.

Many cases and questions have followed from this specific case, and arguments such as these continue to be made and countered. The intersection between law and neuroscience continues to pose controversial and hazy ethical problems in the context of the criminal justice system (Jones et al., 2014). It is clear, however, that adolescent neuroscience and neuropsychological research continue to spill out from the laboratory and into the courts, and it will be interesting to see how society comes to terms with these new discoveries regarding the developing brain, executive function, and culpability.

Adolescent Change in Executive Function Is Neither a Disease nor a Disorder

Although the relationship between poor executive function in teens and dangerous outcomes may seem like a poisonous one, it is important to remember these changes in brain structure and behavior are normative. That is, adolescence should not be viewed as a time of a malfunctioning prefrontal cortex and a misfiring amygdala and striatum that invariably lead to psychological dysfunctions (Casey, Duhoux, & Cohen, 2010). Instead, these neurobehavioral alterations can be viewed as typical and expected, albeit a little scary sometimes (age-related restriction on things like obtaining driver licenses and purchasing and consuming drugs undoubtedly help reduce potential accidents and injuries). It is also worth reiterating that not all teens will show the same temporal patterns of change in executive function and that these changes can be highly dependent on an individual's age, sex, hormones levels, and peers. Finally, it's important to remember that adolescence is not a disorder that needs to be treated or "cured," nor has anyone died of adolescence per se. The majority of adolescent individuals navigate these tumultuous transitions in brain and emotional development just fine and end up learning a great deal about their environments and society in the process. At some level, we just may have to white-knuckle it through this journey and appreciate that it is preparing us for our future destinations.

Recommended Reading

Casey, B. J. (2015). Beyond simple models of self-control to circuit-based accounts of adolescent behavior. *Annual Review of Psychology, 66,* 295–319.

Ernst, M. (2014). The triadic model perspective for the study of adolescent motivated behavior. *Brain and Cognition, 89,* 104–111.

Steinberg, L. (2014). *Age of opportunity: Lessons from the new science of adolescence.* New York, NY: Houghton Mifflin Harcourt.

6

Puberty, Hormones, and the Social Brain

Before we even knew such a thing existed, there was scientific evidence for a diffusible, blood-borne chemical signal (i.e., a hormone) from the gonads that exerts robust influences on behavior. Arnold Berthold conducted the first experiment in behavioral endocrinology in the mid-19th century, in which he found that if a young cockerel was castrated, then his name changed to capon and his wattles and combs failed to develop normally. Moreover, he neither crowed nor displayed the aggressive and sexual behaviors that are characteristic of an adult rooster (Quiring, 1944). The key follow-up experiment showed that if the testes of the cockerel (or testes from a different rooster for that matter) were transplanted back into the body cavity of the capon, then comb, wattle, and behavior all developed normally. Berthold surmised that the testes secrete a substance that normally influences the development of male-typical secondary sex characteristics and behavior. Although he couldn't have come up with the site or mechanism of action of the putative hormone at that time, it now seems obvious that hormonal effects on behaviors as complex as crowing, fighting, and sex would almost have to be through actions in the central nervous system. He also did not know, because he didn't do the experiment, that had he waited until adulthood to re-implant the testes into a rooster castrated at a young age, he would not have observed restoration of those masculine features and behaviors. Such a finding would have likely led him to the conclusion that for permanent masculinizing effects of testicular hormones to occur, exposure to those hormones must happen during a sensitive period earlier in development.

It wasn't until more than 100 years later that Phoenix, Goy, Gerall, and Young (1959) demonstrated that female guinea pigs, if exposed to testosterone during gestation, were both masculinized (more likely to show male-like mounting behavior) and defeminized (less likely to show lordosis or female-like receptive behavior) in adulthood. Furthermore, testosterone treatment of female guinea pigs at later postnatal ages or in adulthood did not result in masculinized or defeminized sexual behaviors. Phoenix et al. reasoned that these early developmental effects of testicular hormones on later adult behavior must be based on permanent, "organizational" effects of these hormones on the structure of the developing nervous system. They went on to speculate that these organizational effects on brain structure effectively program adult behavioral responses to be activated by gonadal hormones later in life. These "activational" effects refer to the ability of gonadal hormones to modify, right then and there, the activity of target cells in ways that facilitate behavior in specific social contexts. Activational effects come and go with the waxing and waning of circulating hormones that occur either naturally (e.g., during annual breeding seasons) or experimentally (e.g., the popular remove-gonads-and-replace-hormones approach to behavioral endocrinology). In contrast, organizational effects of gonadal hormones are more of a hit and run: A brief exposure to testosterone permanently affects developmental trajectory, and there is no need for the hormone to hang around once the deed is done.

With publication of Phoenix et al. (1959), the classic organizational-activational hypothesis of sexual differentiation of behavior was born, and it has been a work in progress ever since. As originally conceived, the organizational-activational hypothesis worked like this: A transient rise in testosterone during perinatal development permanently masculinizes and defeminizes neural circuits in males, while the absence of testosterone in females results in development of a feminine neural phenotype. Upon gonadal maturation during puberty, testicular and ovarian hormones activate previously sexually differentiated circuits to facilitate expression of sex-typical behaviors when and where appropriate. The hypothesis was refined by scores of experiments in the 1960s and 1970s that identified a maximally sensitive period for hormone-dependent sexual differentiation occurring during late prenatal and/or early neonatal development (reviewed in Baum, 1979; Wallen & Baum, 2002). This research led to the corollary hypothesis that the role of gonadal hormones secreted during puberty is purely to activate the previously organized circuits to facilitate the sex-typical expression of physiology and behavior in adulthood.

Another tenet derived from research conducted in this area was that testicular hormones drive the process of creating sexual dimorphisms in nervous system structure. This principle was based in large part on experiments showing that either pharmacological blockade or surgical removal of testicular hormonal influences during the perinatal period was sufficient to prevent both masculinization and defeminization of sexually dimorphic hypothalamic brain regions (reviewed in Cooke, Hegstrom, Villeneuve, &

Breedlove, 1998). In contrast, removal of the ovaries immediately after birth did not have robust consequences on sexual differentiation, and indeed, ovarian hormones are not secreted at this time (Cooke et al., 1998). These studies led to the idea that, in the absence of testicular hormones, the "default" phenotype is essentially female, and ovarian hormones are not actively involved in sexual differentiation of the nervous system.

These long-held canons gradually eroded with the realization that things aren't so simple. We now know that a second wave of sexual differentiation occurs during adolescent development, thanks to the pubertal rise in gonadal hormones. In retrospect, it should have come as no surprise that the metamorphosis of the adolescent brain would be subject to hormonal influences that contribute to the emergence of sex differences during the transition from childhood to adulthood. On an even more basic theoretical level, John Paul Scott, who was studying attachment and socialization in puppies in the 1960s and 1970s, recognized that development comprises multiple sensitive periods during which the nervous system is progressively shaped by experience (which includes internal as well as external signals). Furthermore, he acknowledged that each sensitive period is a commitment to a particular developmental trajectory, limiting the range of possibilities during the succeeding sensitive period (Scott, Stewart, & De Ghett, 1974). Scott also noted that sensitive periods occur during times of rapid or high rate of change, and puberty certainly falls into that category. We also now know that ovarian hormones acting during puberty play an active role in the further sexual differentiation of brain and behavior. That is, during adolescence there appears to be ovarian hormone-dependent, active feminization, and thus, the female phenotype may not be a passive, "default" outcome as originally proposed.

Here, we will specifically focus on hormone-dependent organization of social behaviors during puberty and adolescence. Social behavior is by no means the only type of behavior that is susceptible to permanent shaping by pubertal hormones. However, there are more examples of pubertal organization of social behaviors than any other category of behavior, and most of these examples are of *male* social behaviors. This may be because adult social behaviors are almost always sexually differentiated and activated by gonadal hormones and therefore are the low-hanging fruit for study of behaviors subject to further organization during puberty. It may also be a function of the importance that adolescent maturation of social behaviors has played in evolution, namely the evolutionary pressure to enhance reproductive fitness, particularly in males. Either way, the focus of this chapter will be on social behaviors, although later in the chapter we'll highlight some examples of other categories of behavior that are organized by gonadal hormones during puberty and adolescence.

Social Cognition and Social Reorientation During Adolescence

Luckily, conceptual frameworks exist for considering social behaviors in the context of motivated behaviors, for how social cognition influences the expression of these behaviors, and for how social cognition is transformed during puberty and adolescence. Research in these areas has also been facilitated by the recently coined notion of the *social brain*. We will first look at some of these frameworks and then, where possible, map research on the adolescent organization of social behaviors onto these theoretical constructs.

Let us start by operationally defining social cognition as the mental processes by which an individual encodes, interprets, and responds to sensory information from an animal of the same species (Adolphs, 2001; Dodge, 1993). As simple as that may sound, personal experiences tell us that social cognition is anything but. The encoding of primary sensory stimuli from another animal is relatively straightforward, but how that sensory information is then perceived and interpreted is a function of an individual's sex, age, social experience, and, for humans, culture. Interpretation of a social stimulus usually involves assignment of positive or negative valence along with some associated emotional state, which, in turn, leads to motivation to approach or avoid the perceived stimulus, and, finally, selection of a behavioral response. Here, an individual may have a number of different possible behavioral reactions to evaluate and choose from. The outcome of the social interaction influences the probability that the chosen behavioral response will be selected again in the future. That is, individuals learn to modify their behavior based on positive or negative outcomes of their social experiences, and these behavioral adaptations lead to social proficiency and social competence.

Research on social cognition inevitably led to the birth of social neuroscience, which is the investigation of the neurobiological basis of social cognition. Naturally, it did not take long for social neuroscience to invoke the concept of the social brain in reference to those neural circuits that link perception of social stimuli with emotion and motivated behavior, including behavioral flexibility. Functional imaging studies in humans and markers

of neuronal activation in non-human animals, along with lesion and pharmacological approaches, have identified a collection of interconnected brain
regions called the social information processing network (SIPN), which
includes sensory association cortex, the extended amygdala, hypothalamus, prefrontal cortex, and dorsal and ventral striatum (Nelson, Leibenluft,
McClure, & Pine, 2005).

An important conceptual framework for thinking about the maturation
of social behavior and social cognition during puberty and adolescence is
social reorientation, which refers to the periadolescent shift from family to
peers as the primary focus of social interactions (Nelson et al., 2005). Social
reorientation necessarily requires remodeling of the SIPN because the relative valence and motivational salience of family and peers essentially flip-
flops over the course of puberty and adolescence and, with that, a completely
new suite of behavioral adaptations must be learned. The SIPN as originally
conceived in the context of social reorientation comprises three functionally
distinct components: the sensory detection node, the affective node, and the
cognitive-regulatory node. The job of the detection node is to recognize and
categorize sensory stimuli as social. Once a social stimulus is detected, then
the affective node assigns an emotional quality and motivational salience to
it. Finally, the social stimulus is processed by the cognitive-regulatory node,
which has the complicated task of assessing the mental state of the other animal from which the social stimulus is derived, inhibiting potentially maladaptive behaviors, and generating adaptive and goal-directed behaviors.

The framers of the social reorientation model of the SIPN proposed that
the detection mode matured early in life (e.g., even very young children are
capable of distinguishing social from nonsocial stimuli), and it did not really undergo a major overhaul during adolescence. In contrast, the affective
node, which includes the amygdala and other limbic regions, was proposed
to be significantly affected by the pubertal rise in gonadal hormones, as these
regions are chock-full of receptors for these hormones. Lastly, the cognitive-
regulatory node, which includes areas of the prefrontal cortex, matures relatively late, as the structural magnetic resonance imaging studies of human
brains have shown (see Chapter 4). Because adolescent maturation of this
node is not particularly temporally correlated with the onset of puberty and
hormone secretion, it was proposed that development of this node is not as
susceptible to hormonal influences as the affective node (although we now
know that hormones do influence adolescent maturation of this node; see
Chapter 4 and later in this chapter). Finally, because part of its function is

to allow behavioral adaptations in response to social experience, maturation of the cognitive-regulatory node was proposed to be relatively slow and
iterative. (Readers may note that the feature of a late-maturing cognitive-
regulatory node in the SIPN is also a feature of the triadic model of adolescent
maturation of decision-making described in Chapter 5.) This conceptualiza-
tion of adolescent maturation of the SIPN in the context of social reorientation is a useful heuristic for research that can experimentally investigate the
neurobiology of social reorientation in animal models. So let us try to merge
the behavioral components of social cognition with components of the social
brain and look at them through the lens of time as the process of social reorientation unfolds.

As previously alluded to, social information processing theory (aka social
cognition) outlines a sequence of mental processes leading up to the expression of social behavior. Again, these are as follows:

1. *Encoding* of the sensory aspects of a social stimulus or cue. Social
   stimuli are often complex and include multiple sensory modalities,
   and with social experience, the encoding process is refined so that
   an individual selectively attends to particular features of the social stimulus, presumably those that offer the most socially relevant
   information.
2. *Mental representation* of the social stimulus, which essentially boils
   down to how the stimulus is perceived. In this process, meaning, emotion, and valence are assigned to the stimulus.
3. *Response accessing and evaluation* is the mental representation of an
   internal list of the various behaviors that could be chosen to respond
   to the social stimulus. Not all of these responses are a good idea, however, and the individual must figure out which responses could lead to
   a bad outcome and which could lead to a good outcome, scratching
   the former off the list and retaining the latter. Of the responses that potentially lead to a good outcome, one is selected that seems best in the
   moment.
4. *Enactment* is the overt behavioral expression of the selected response.

We have to incorporate what psychologists refer to as *theory of mind* into this
social information processing framework. During mental representation, an
individual has to make a best guess as to what the social stimulus conveys
about the other animal's intent and motivation. Then, during response

evaluation, one has to predict how the other individual is likely to react to the response that is ultimately enacted.

Although these processes are sequential with respect to a single stimulus, the reality is that the social interaction is dynamic, so that new stimuli may show up before enactment of the behavioral response to the original stimulus. The dynamics of a social interaction thus require constant stimulus reassessment and response re-evaluation. Moreover, not only must many social graces be practiced to be effective, but also we have to rely on experience to teach us which behavioral responses are a good idea in a particular social context. Thus, social cognition is of necessity an iterative process that is sculpted by development *and* experience.

Returning to the focus of this chapter on the hormonal organization of social behaviors during adolescence, it is helpful to consider whether or not these concepts of social cognition can be probed in laboratory animal models. To start with, how an animal perceives a social stimulus, and whether or not the stimulus is rewarding or aversive, is relatively easy to assess. One can use a simple preference test to determine how much time an animal spends in the vicinity of two different conspecifics or sensory stimuli emanating from them. Conditioned place preference (CPP) tests indicate whether a social stimulus is rewarding by determining whether an animal prefers to spend more time in a test chamber that has been paired with the stimulus compared to a test chamber that has not been paired with the stimulus. Similarly, conditioned place avoidance tests can determine whether a stimulus is perceived as aversive. The reinforcing value or incentive salience of a stimulus can also be assessed through instrumental tasks; that is, will an animal work (e.g., press a lever) to gain access to the stimulus, and, if so, just how hard will they work for it? The next process in social cognition—evaluation of potential behavioral responses—is not as easy to investigate in animals, because we cannot know the cognitive routes an animal takes to mull over the pros and cons of a particular response. The best we can do is to observe the response that happens and infer that, for whatever reason, the animal deemed this response to be the best idea under the circumstances. Then, by experimentally manipulating the quality and quantity of experience that the animal has with that stimulus, we can assess whether or not the animal makes adjustments in its response to the stimulus over time. Monitoring behavioral adaptations to social experience gives an indication of behavioral flexibility and social proficiency. Therefore, although it is possible to probe most aspects of social cognition in laboratory animals, these models are extremely limited in their usefulness to study theory of mind. With these caveats about the strengths and limitations of animal models in investigating social cognition, let's see what can be learned from them to understand which aspects of social reorientation are organized by gonadal hormones during puberty and adolescence.

Experimental Paradigms for Assessing
Organizational Effects of Gonadal Hormones

Many of the examples of organization of behavior by pubertal hormones were identified using an experimental approach that is in many respects is similar to the one used by Berthold in his early experiments on developing roosters: remove and replace. That is, if you want to know what testicular hormones are doing to brain and behavior during the pubertal period, well then, take the testes out just before the start of puberty and see what happens. Next, to confirm that whatever did (or didn't) happen in the absence of the testes was due to the absence of testosterone in particular, you remove the testes just before puberty, and this time give back testosterone, and see what happens. Berthold did this by reimplanting either the testes he had just removed or the testes from another rooster. Remember, he had no idea there was such a thing as testosterone, and his goal was simply to determine whether there was *something* about the testes that imparted the masculine traits he was looking at.

These days, we can specifically replace testosterone (or other testicular hormones of interest), usually via implants designed to release the hormone over a period of weeks to months. To determine whether puberty is a particularly sensitive period of development for organizational actions of testosterone, it is necessary to manipulate *the age* at which testosterone replacement is performed. Furthermore, the experimental design has to be one that permits dissociation of activational effects of testosterone from organizational effects of testosterone. To illustrate the decision tree underlying this type of investigation, we'll draw on experiments we have used in the male Syrian hamster to dissect out activational from organizational effects of testosterone on social behaviors during pubertal maturation (reviewed in Schulz & Sisk, 2016; Sisk, 2016). The first step is to compare the behavior of juvenile males with that of adult males during social interactions. If juvenile and adult behaviors are different, either quantitatively or qualitatively, then we ask whether pubertal hormones are involved in adolescent maturation of the behavior. To answer this question, the remove-and-replace strategy is used in subsequent experiments: Juvenile hamsters are castrated, hormone is immediately replaced, and social behavior is examined while the hamsters are still juvenile. If testosterone-treated juveniles display adult-like behavior, then one can conclude that activational effects of testosterone alone are sufficient for expression of the adult behavioral phenotype. If testosterone fails to activate the behavior in juveniles, then the conclusion is that further neural maturation during adolescence is required before activational effects can occur, and this additional maturation may or may not depend on organizational effects of testosterone during puberty (Figure 6.1; Table 6.1).

To assess the organizational effects of pubertal testosterone (or one of its metabolites) on the maturation of social cognition, male hamsters are deprived of testosterone via removal of the testes either during puberty or for an equivalent amount of time in adulthood, and then social interactions are assessed after 1 to 2 weeks of testosterone replacement. Given the specifics of these experimental manipulations, we refer to the group with no testes/testosterone present during puberty as NoT@P and those with testes/testosterone present during puberty as T@P. Although these shorthand versions of these group names are a bit clunky, writing them out every time is even clunkier, so please forgive the literary license. With this jargon in mind, if the previously described experiment was conducted and the behavior of NoT@P and T@P males differed, then adult-typical expression of the behavior depends on organizational effects of pubertal testosterone.

Pubertal Organization of Male Sexual Behavior: Lessons From the Syrian Hamster

The Syrian hamster, *Mesocricetus auratus* (aka the golden hamster—sold in pet stores), has taught us many lessons about the neurobiology of social behaviors, including sexual and agonistic behaviors. Oddly enough, Syrian hamsters are not social creatures by nature. In the wild, they live in solitary burrows and tolerate each other peacefully only during sexual encounters. Adult females are up to 25% larger than adult males, and females are clearly in charge when it comes to mating: Female hamsters are receptive to advances from a male on only 1 day of her 4-day estrous cycle. If Syrian hamsters are not particularly social, as defined by seeking out each other's company, then

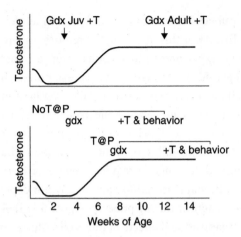

Figure 6.1. Experimental strategy for determining activation or pubertal organization of male behavior by testosterone.

Top panel: If the behavior of castrated and testosterone-treated juveniles (Juv+T) is similar to that of castrated and testosterone-treated adults (Adult+T), then we infer that the behavior is activated by the pubertal rise in testosterone and its expression requires no additional maturational process. Bottom panel: If testosterone does not activate the behavior in juvenile males, then the NoT@P (no testes/testosterone at puberty) paradigm is used to assess whether testosterone organizes the behavior during puberty. Behavior is compared in males that were gonadectomized before (NoT@P) or after (T@P) puberty and then given testosterone replacement several weeks later, when both groups are in young adulthood. If testosterone replacement fails to activate behavior in NoT@P males but does activate behavior in T@P males, then we infer that the presence of testosterone during puberty and adolescence organizes behavioral circuits and programs the quantity or quality of activational responses to hormone in adulthood.

what makes them a good species for studying hormonal influences on the development of social behavior? Well, just because hamsters do not live in social groups and adults do not typically display affiliative behaviors, this does not mean they do not engage in social behaviors, as defined by interactions between two animals of the same species. Sex and aggression are both social behaviors, and hamsters are very good at both.

As far as sex goes, one feature of male hamster sexual behavior that is different from that of other commonly studied laboratory rodents (e.g., rats and mice) is the utter dependence of the behavior on neural processing of

Table 6.1. How to Determine Whether Adult Male Behavior Is Organized by Pubertal Actions of Testosterone

Behavioral comparison	Conclusion
Juvenile = Adult	Behavior doesn't require pubertal maturation. End of story.
Juvenile ≠ Adult	Behavior requires pubertal maturation. Proceed with remove and replace experiments.
Juvenile + T = Adult + T	Behavior is activated at puberty by testosterone. End of story.
Juvenile + T ≠ Adult + T	Behavior requires either hormone-dependent or -independent organization during puberty. Proceed with NoT@P experiments.
NoT@P = T@P	Behavior doesn't require pubertal organization by testosterone.
NoT@P ≠ T@P	Behavior is organized at puberty by testosterone.

female pheromones present in vaginal secretions (VS; Wood, 1998; Wood & Newman, 1995). For example, if the olfactory bulbs are removed from a sexually experienced adult male hamster, he will no longer mate with a receptive female, even though his testosterone levels are sufficient to activate the behavior. This provides an opportunity to investigate mechanisms of neural integration of external sensory and internal hormonal stimuli that together regulate sexual behavior.

Our own research program has relied heavily on male Syrian hamsters for unveiling some general principles about hormonal organization of social information processing and the social brain. Our initial investigations, begun in the late 1990s, focused on the role of testicular hormones in the pubertal maturation of male sexual behavior. Here, we employed the remove-and-replace strategy, this time doing the experiment in both juvenile and adult hamsters. We found that male sexual behavior cannot be activated in gonadectomized juvenile male hamsters by treating them with either testosterone or its biologically active metabolites estradiol and dihydrotestosterone, even though the same treatments reliably activate sexual behavior in adults (Meek, Romeo, Novak, & Sisk, 1997; Romeo, Cook-Wiens, Richardson, & Sisk, 2001; Romeo, Wagner, Jansen, Diedrich, & Sisk, 2002). Our initial hypothetical explanation to explain this finding was that perhaps the juvenile hamster brain does not express sufficient levels of steroid hormone receptors, the intracellular proteins that when activated by hormones collaborate with other transcription factors in the cell nucleus to influence gene expression, protein synthesis, cell metabolism, excitability, and, ultimately, behavior. To test this hypothesis, we compared three different cellular markers of steroid hormone receptor activation in the brain in juvenile and adult male hamsters, predicting that if the hypothesis was correct, then the responses of adults to hormone treatment would be of greater magnitude than those of juveniles. The three responses studied were (a) upregulation of androgen receptor (AR) by testosterone and dihydrotestosterone; (b) upregulation of aromatase activity by testosterone (aromatase is the enzyme that converts testosterone to estradiol); and (c) upregulation of progesterone receptor by estradiol. In all three cases, we found that the responses of juvenile hamsters following hormone treatment were at least as great as those in adults, sometimes even greater (Romeo, Diedrich, & Sisk, 2000; Romeo et al., 2001, 2002; Romeo, Wade, Venier, & Sisk, 1999). Therefore, at the level of the cell, we had no evidence that decreased hormone receptor availability or change in receptor function explained the inability of hormones to activate sexual behavior in juveniles.

We then turned to the other essential element for male sexual behavior in hamsters—neural processing of female pheromones. If steroid hormones are doing their thing in the juvenile brain, perhaps what was missing was the ability of juvenile males to perceive female pheromones as a socio-sexual stimulus. At the time, several different laboratories were investigating neural processing of female chemosensory stimuli in male hamsters, and it was the conventional wisdom that female pheromones induced a characteristic pattern of neuronal activation in the male hamster brain, as reflected in induced expression of the immediate early gene c-Fos. So, we set out to compare the neural activation pattern induced by female pheromones in juvenile and adult males, focusing on the cell groups that had already been identified as responders to pheromones in adults, namely the medial amygdala, bed nucleus of the stria terminalis, and medial preoptic area. Much to our surprise, the c-Fos response to female pheromones in these cell groups was indistinguishable between juvenile and adult males (Romeo, Parfitt, Richardson, & Sisk, 1998), suggesting that neural processing of female pheromones in juvenile males was already adult-like and didn't even require adult levels of testosterone to be observed.

Although frustrated with our inability to answer this experimental question, we starting thinking about sexual behavior within the framework of social cognition and social reorientation. We became intrigued by the possibility that social reorientation may involve a transition in social reward; that is, peers become more socially rewarding than they were before, eventually out-rewarding even family members as the preferred social realm. Going back to the question of why testosterone-treated juvenile male hamsters won't mate with a receptive female, perhaps it is the case that female pheromones are perceived as female alright, but if you are still a juvenile, so what? Sexual interactions with that large (and sometimes aggressive) female may not be enticing, and, in particular, those female pheromones that are so critical for expression of adult male sexual behavior may simply not constitute a social reward in juveniles. We had known for some time that gonad-intact adult male hamsters prefer female pheromones to other odors and that this preference emerges during puberty (Johnston & Coplin, 1979). This led us to test the idea that the expression of sexual behavior occurs only in adulthood because the sensory stimuli necessary for the behavior only become rewarding once some maturational process has happened during puberty and adolescence.

To test this hypothesis, we turned to the CPP assay, a commonly used test to judge whether a particular stimulus or experience is rewarding to an animal. The CPP test takes advantage of the fact that animals learn to associate places with rewards. It employs a classical conditioning paradigm in which an unconditioned stimulus (a stimulus that is inherently rewarding, no learning required) is repeatedly paired with a particular context that is distinctly different from another context in which the animal never experiences the unconditioned stimulus. If after conditioning the animal prefers to be in the context that was paired with the unconditioned stimulus, then we infer that the unconditioned stimulus was rewarding, and the associated context has acquired conditioned stimulus status. In our case, we wanted to determine whether female pheromones, by themselves, could serve as an unconditioned stimulus for formation of a CPP in juvenile and adult male hamsters. In our version of the CPP test, we used a three-chamber apparatus in which the two outer chambers were different in floor texture and odor (Figure 6.2A). After a habituation period, we determined which chamber a hamster preferred to spent most of its time. Then, the initially nonpreferred chamber was paired with a vial containing VS (the female pheromones) over a series of conditioning days, while on alternate days the initially preferred chamber was paired with an empty vial. Formation of a CPP is defined by a change in preference for the initially nonpreferred chamber after conditioning, as evidenced by a significant change in a preference score determined before and after conditioning.

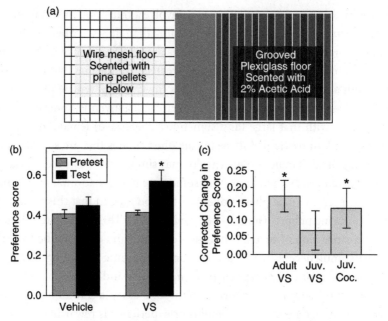

Figure 6.2. Conditioned place preference (CPP). (a) Three-chamber apparatus used for conditioned place preference. (b) Mean (± standard error of the mean) preference score on pretest (gray bars) and test (black bars) for control and vaginal secretions (VS) groups. Asterisk indicates that adult male hamsters form a CPP for the compartment associated with female odors (significant change in preference score between pretest and test, $p < 0.05$). (c) Corrected change in preference scores when tested for a CPP for VS and cocaine. Adult males showed a CPP for VS, whereas juvenile males did not; however, juvenile males did show a CPP for cocaine. Asterisks indicate a significant difference between corrected change in preference score and 0.00 within a group ($p < 0.05$). Adapted and reprinted from M. R. Bell, S. H. Meerts, & C. L. Sisk, 2010, Male Syrian hamsters demonstrate a conditioned place preference for sexual behavior and female chemosensory stimuli, *Hormones and Behavior, 58,* 410–414, and M. R. Bell, K. C. De Lorme, R. J. Figueira, D. Kashy, & C. L. Sisk, 2013, Adolescent gain in positive valence of a socially relevant stimulus: Engagement of the mesocorticolimbic reward circuitry, *European Journal of Neuroscience, 37,* 457–468. Used with permission from Elsevier and John Wiley and Sons, Inc.

Sexually inexperienced adults readily form a CPP for VS, as shown by the significant change in preference score after pairing the initially nonpreferred chamber with VS (Bell, Meerts, & Sisk, 2010; Figure 6.2B). In contrast, pre-pubertal males do not form a CPP to VS, even though they form a CPP to cocaine, indicating they are capable of forming a CPP (Bell, De Lorme, Figueira, Kashy, & Sisk, 2013; Figure 6.2C). These initial studies told us that female pheromones are an unconditioned social reward to adult male hamsters, but to juveniles, not so much. Based on these results, we hypothesized that social reorientation, the shift in focus of social interactions from kin to unrelated peers, involves a switch in the salience and rewarding properties of social stimuli. Put another way, juvenile male hamsters are, at best, indifferent to the odors of a receptive female, but something happens during puberty and adolescence to make this chemosensory stimulus attractive and rewarding, at least to an adult male hamster's way of thinking.

Applying the experimental strategy outlined in Figure 6.1 and Table 6.1, we determined that testosterone, independent of age, *activates* the perception of female pheromones as rewarding. First, gonadectomized, testosterone-treated juveniles formed a CPP to VS, just like gonadectomized, testosterone-treated adults (Bell & Sisk, 2013; Figure 6.3). Second, neither gonadectomized juveniles nor gonadectomized adults formed a CPP without testosterone replacement (Bell & Sisk, 2013; Figure 6.3). Third, both NoT@P and T@P males form a CPP to female pheromones if replaced with testosterone in adulthood, so no additional maturational processes during puberty and adolescence are required for VS to be perceived as rewarding by adult males (De Lorme, Bell, & Sisk, 2012). Apparently, all that is needed is some testosterone, at any time, for this remarkable transformation to take place.

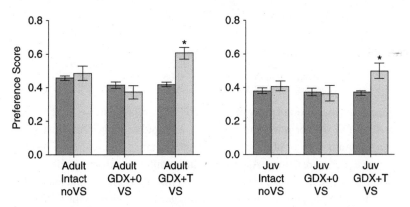

Figure 6.3. Conditioned place preference (CPP) in gonadectomized hamsters. If gonadectomized and treated with vehicle, neither adult (left panel) nor juvenile (right panel) male hamsters form a CPP to female pheromones. If gonadectomized and treated with testosterone, both adult and juvenile male hamsters form a CPP to female pheromones.

How does testosterone do that? At this point, we do not know the full story, but it appears to involve activation of dopamine receptors. Specifically, we found that a systemic injection of the dopamine receptor antagonist haloperidol given to testosterone-treated juvenile males just prior to the conditioning sessions (i.e., on those days when the male spends time in the chamber with the VS) prevents formation of the CPP (Bell & Sisk, 2013; Figure 6.4).

Where does testosterone do that? When the *c*-Fos response to female pheromones is examined in gonad intact male hamsters, we find that this social sensory stimulus elicits comparable increases in *c*-Fos activity in various forebrain regions, like the medial amygdala, stria terminalis, preoptic area, and the dopamine neurons of the ventral tegmental area (VTA) of both juveniles and adults (Bell, De Lorme, et al., 2013; Romeo et al., 1998). The medial amygdala receives direct input from the olfactory bulb, so the fact that the *c*-Fos response to female pheromones in this region is similar in juveniles and adults is evidence that (a) juveniles do detect this stimulus and (b) initial central processing of the stimulus is likely the same in juveniles and adults.

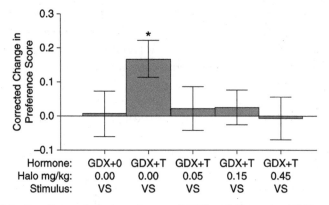

Figure 6.4. Conditioned place preference (CPP) and dopamine. CPP to vaginal secretions (VS) in hormone and dopamine manipulated juvenile hamsters. Mean (± standard error of the mean) corrected changes in preference and difference scores are shown. Asterisks indicate difference from no change (0.0 on the *y*-axis). Testosterone treatment in juvenile hamsters facilitated an adult-like CPP for VS, and dopamine receptor antagonism prevented the CPP for VS at multiple doses of haloperidol. Adapted and reprinted from Bell & Sisk, 2013, Dopamine mediates testosterone-induced social reward in male Syrian hamsters. *Endocrinology, 154,* 1225–1234. Used with permission from Oxford University Press.

However, downstream central processing of pheromones must differ at the two ages, because we know that female pheromones are an unconditioned reward in adults, but not juveniles. Indeed, only in adults is there an increase in c-Fos levels in the VTA and nucleus accumbens, indicating that adolescent maturation of social reward engages the mesocorticolimbic reward circuitry (Bell, De Lorme et al., 2013).

Since testosterone treatment of juvenile males is sufficient for them to form a CPP to female odors (Bell & Sisk, 2013), we next determined whether testosterone-treated juveniles would show a c-Fos response to female odors that was similar to that of adult males. We did not find this to be the case; female odors elicited a response in VTA in adults only (Bell, Meerts, & Sisk, 2013). Thus, even though testosterone activates formation of a CPP to female odors in juvenile males, it does not recapitulate the adult c-Fos response to female odors in the mesocorticolimibc reward circuitry, leading to the conclusion that the adult response to female odors in these brain regions reflects both activational and organizational effects of pubertal testosterone.

All of this is well and good, but we still have not figured out what keeps those juvenile males, even if bathed in testosterone, from mating with a female. Maybe they are simply afraid of her (remember she is the larger one). We do not think that some sort of neural organization by testosterone during puberty is the answer, because male hamsters that have not experienced testosterone during the normal time of puberty will mate with a receptive female after testosterone replacement in adulthood. On the surface, then, the overt activation of male sexual behavior by testosterone in adulthood does not require hormone-dependent organization. However, the behavior of NoT@P males is decidedly not the same as that of T@P males. For example, absolute amounts of reproductive behavior are lower than those of T@P males, and these behavioral deficits in NoT@P males persist after a prolonged period of testosterone replacement in adulthood, and even with sexual experience (Schulz et al., 2004). Based on these behavioral findings, we postulated that one or more aspect of social cognition was organized by pubertal testosterone, and our next line of investigation set out to determine which ones were impaired in NoT@P males. Our earlier experiments on social reward had already shown that NoT@P males form a CPP to either a receptive female or her odors, so the perception (mental representation) of female pheromones as a rewarding social stimulus does not depend on hormone-dependent organization during puberty. Further, we haven't detected deficits in the performance of mating behaviors per se in NoT@P males; that is, enactment of these behaviors does not appear to be problematic for them. What does appear to be problematic is their ability to make the appropriate behavioral adaptations after social experience: NoT@P males do not compare favorably with T@P males when it comes to social proficiency or competence.

What is the evidence that social proficiency depends on organizing effects of pubertal testosterone? Well, if the behavior of NoT@P and T@P males is monitored across a series of either male–female or male–male social interactions, it turns out that the T@P males make behavioral adaptations that are typical of socially experienced gonad-intact male hamsters, whereas the NoT@P males do not. Let's take male–female social interactions and experience first. Sexually naïve, gonadally intact adult male hamsters normally display high levels of ectopic (misdirected) mounts during their first encounter with a receptive female. With sexual experience, however, ectopic mounts decrease to low levels and, thereafter, happen only occasionally. T@P male hamsters also show this behavioral adaptation to experience, but NoT@P hamsters do not (De Lorme & Sisk, 2016; Schulz & Sisk, 2006; Figure 6.5).

Another example of social proficiency in hamsters can be seen over the course of repeated male–male social interactions. During the first encounter between two unfamiliar males in a neutral arena, an aggressive interaction initially occurs, and then a dominant-subordinate relationship is typically established within a few minutes. During subsequent encounters, there is little frank aggression. Instead, the dominant–subordinate relationship is maintained through benign chemosensory communication accomplished by the deposition of secretions from flank glands. Although both the dominant and subordinate male display flank-marking behavior, the frequency of flank marking is much higher in the dominant male compared to the subordinate (Ferris, Axelson, Shinto, & Albers, 1987). We found that this pattern of social proficiency, in which overt aggression is replaced by nonlife threatening flank marking to keep the peace, is not seen in NoT@P males. NoT@P males are somewhat less likely to form a dominant-subordinate relationship in the first place. Nevertheless, when they do form a relationship, both the dominant and subordinate NoT@P males display lower levels of flank marking than do T@P males. Moreover, if a pair of NoT@P males that have formed a dominant–subordinate relationship are reintroduced the next day, they end up duking it out again instead of using flank marks to remind each other who's dominant (De Lorme & Sisk, 2013).

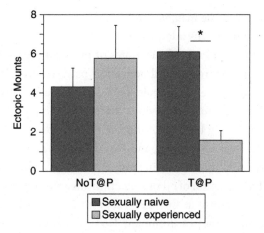

Figure 6.5. Interaction between sexual experience and adolescent testicular hormone exposure. Males exposed to testicular hormones during pubertal development (T@P) display significantly fewer incorrectly oriented (ectopic) mounts with repeated sexual experience. In contrast, males deprived of pubertal testicular hormones (NoT@P) do not improve their mounting accuracy with repeated sexual experience. Asterisk indicates $p < 0.05$. Reprinted from K. M. Schulz & C. L. Sisk, 2006, Pubertal hormones, the adolescent brain, and the maturation of social behaviors: Lessons from the Syrian hamster, *Molecular and Cellular Endocrinology, 254–255*, 120–126. Used with permission from Elsevier.

So, it appears that NoT@P males lack some basic social skills, and exposure to testicular hormones during adolescence is sufficient to program these skills. It is not presently clear what exactly is impaired in NoT@P males and why they don't seem to be able to learn from experience. It could be a simple case of poor memory of previous social interactions, but if that were all there is to it, then you might expect NoT@P males to take a long time to form a CPP to female odors, which they don't. Furthermore, latencies to engage in mating behavior decrease with sexual experience in NoT@P males, so they appear to be remembering something. Other possibilities are that NoT@P males have poor impulse control, are inflexible, or perseverate even when the behavior is ultimately maladaptive. We tend to lean toward interpretations that involve some sort of impairment in executive function when testicular hormones are not around to organize the relevant corticolimbic circuits during adolescent development. And because impulse control, habits, and behavioral flexibility involve different components of executive function circuitry, pinpointing the precise nature of the behavioral deficits in NoT@P males will provide some insight into which parts of the circuitry are organized by testosterone during adolescence.

To identify potential neural substrates of pubertal organization of social proficiency, we compared neural activation patterns in T@P and NoT@P male hamsters after a series of male–male social interactions (De Lorme & Sisk, 2013). Recall from our previous discussion that NoT@P males show atypical flank-marking behavior, whether they are the dominant or subordinate individual within the pair, and NoT@P males appear to rely on overt aggression instead of flank marking to maintain the dominant–subordinate relationship. Examination of c-Fos induction after an agonistic encounter revealed that the response in the lateral septum is greater in dominant T@P males compared to that of dominant NoT@P males. Notably, the lateral septum suppresses aggression (Albert & Walsh, 1984; David, Cervantes, Trosky, Salinas, & Delville, 2004) and is involved in regulating flank marking (Ferris, Gold, De Vries, & Potegal, 1990; Irvin et al., 1990). Therefore, organizational effects of pubertal testosterone might be required to engage the lateral septum to promote socially proficient male–male interactions.

To summarize, our studies on the role of testosterone in adolescent maturation of male social cognition and behavior provide two basic take-home messages. First, during the process of social reorientation, when the focus of social interactions switches from family to peers, social stimuli take on new meaning and motivational properties, and this shift in social reward is an outcome of *activational* effects of testosterone during puberty. Second, the adolescent gain in social proficiency, which is the capacity to adapt based on one's social experience, is an outcome of *organizational* effects of testosterone during puberty. Testosterone is definitely multitasking during puberty and adolescence.

Generalization to Males of Other Mammalian Species

You have just read a very specific story about testosterone and the pubertal programming of social cognition and social behaviors in male Syrian hamsters. All well and good, but do things generally work the same way in males of other species? And what about other types of behavior? Is there hormonal programming of them during puberty as well? Of course, the answer is no. And you wouldn't expect that to be the case, given vast species differences in the social world in which individuals live and the types of behaviors that are ultimately important for reproductive fitness for a given species. However, there is evidence that testicular hormones, acting during the time of puberty, do organize an assortment of neural circuits and behaviors in a variety of species (Schulz & Sisk, 2016), which we turn to next.

Pubertal Testosterone and the Programming of Other Behaviors

Let us first consider anxiety. Anxiety may seem like an out-of-the-blue transition from pubertal organization of male social behaviors to pubertal programing of other behaviors, but it so happens that anxiety-like behavior in rats is the original example of how testicular hormones, acting during puberty, program sex differences in behavior. It turns out that adult male rats walk around less than female rats when tested in an open-field arena (a commonly used behavioral test to assess anxiety-like behavior in rodents), suggesting that the open field is more anxiogenic to males than to females. It appears that testicular hormones organize this sex difference in open-field activity during puberty, because prepubertal castration results in increased activity in males in adulthood (Brand & Slob, 1988). Similarly, male–male social interactions are reduced in a novel environment compared with a familiar environment, indicating an anxiogenic effect of the novel environment in males. This effect of the novel environment on male–male social interactions develops during puberty; that is, juvenile male rats do not seem perturbed by a novel environment (Primus & Kellogg, 1989). Prepubertal castration prevents the pubertal emergence of the novel environment effect, yet castration in adulthood does not alter the effect of the novel environment on social interactions, indicating that the novel environment still spooks adult male rats even in the absence of circulating testosterone. The proof that pubertal testosterone programs this anxiety-like behavior comes from experiments in which testosterone replacement to prepubertally castrated rats during the time of puberty, *but not in adulthood*, reinstates the novel environment effect in adulthood (Primus & Kellogg, 1990). Testicular hormones appear to do this by altering the response of the benzodiazepine-GABA receptor complex in neurons to environmental challenge (Primus & Kellogg, 1991). Furthermore, the hormonal agent in charge of this masculinizing effect is not testosterone itself, but its estrogenic metabolite estradiol. We know this because inhibiting activity of the aromatase enzyme throughout puberty in male rats completely prevents the pubertal emergence of the novel environment effect on social interactions, whereas pharmacological blockade of androgen receptor activation throughout puberty does nothing to prevent a novel environment from becoming an anxiety-provoking situation for male rats (Kellogg & Lundin, 1999).

What about behaviors that do not involve interaction with a conspecific? Let's take spatial cognition as an example. On average, men perform better than women in tests of spatial cognition (Maguire, Burgess, & O'Keefe, 1999), and this difference in spatial abilities may be organized by pubertal hormones. Evidence for this comes from a study in which spatial cognition was compared in men with idiopathic hypogonadotropic hypogonadism (IHH) that began before puberty and men with IHH acquired in adulthood (Hier & Crowley, 1982). Remember, IHH is a disorder associated with dysfunctional GnRH secretion (see Chapter 2), and thus the former group had low or undetectable levels of circulating gonadal steroids during the normal time of puberty and adolescence, whereas the latter group experienced typical levels of gonadal hormones during this period. Spatial cognition was impaired in men not exposed to pubertal hormones, both in comparison to healthy control subjects and to men with acquired IHH in adulthood (Hier & Crowley, 1982), suggesting that testicular hormones during puberty organize circuits underlying spatial cognition. Another study of human spatial cognition included women subjects with a variation of congenital adrenal hyperplasia that leads to slightly but chronically elevated levels of adrenal androgens during childhood and early puberty. These women performed better in a virtual Morris Water maze (a test of spatial memory) compared with healthy subjects, again suggesting a pubertal organizational influence of adrenal androgens on spatial ability (Mueller et al., 2008). Notably, spatial memory is dependent on the hippocampus, and synaptic plasticity in the hippocampus appears to be organized by pubertal androgens (Hebbard, King, Malsbury, & Harley, 2003), providing a potential mechanism by which pubertal testosterone could organize hippocampus-dependent learning and memory, including spatial cognition.

It appears, then, that pubertal testosterone (or one of its metabolites) organizes sexual behavior, aggressive behavior, anxiety-like behaviors, and spatial cognition in males, with the caveat that we don't have experimental confirmation that hormonal programming of this wide range of adult behaviors occurs across the board in all species. However, there really is no good reason to expect universal effects of pubertal testosterone on all behaviors in all species. Evolution doesn't work that way. More on this point later, but first let us wrap up this chapter by looking at the organizing effects of ovarian hormones during puberty on female behaviors.

Ovarian Hormones and Organization of the Adolescent Brain

As mentioned earlier, the research on potential organizational effects of ovarian hormones on female behavior has lagged behind the research on testicular hormones and male behavior. There are probably a couple of reasons for this. First is a general reluctance to use female subjects when one is interested in adult behavior of rodents. For decades, researchers have incorrectly presumed that the cyclical nature of hormone secretion in females introduces within-group variability and is just too difficult and expensive to gain experimental control over. Although that notion was recently debunked (Becker, Prendergast, & Liang, 2016; Prendergast, Onishi, & Zucker, 2014), it nevertheless continues to be a deterrent for including females in neurobiological research that isn't deliberately directed toward understanding sex differences or female-specific physiology and behavior. A second, and perhaps more understandable reason for the relative lateness of work on pubertal organization in females, is that the dogma for so long had been that femaleness is the "default" phenotype, and to switch that developmental progression, testosterone must come along and masculinize both somatic tissues and the nervous system. In other words, the female phenotype does not require active feminization by estrogen or any other hormone produced by the female body; it's just what you get in the absence of masculinizing influences of testosterone. In fact, the prevailing view of perinatal sexual differentiation of the rodent nervous system is still just that, so it would be arguably natural to assume that the same principle applies to the second wave of hormone-dependent organization of the brain during puberty and adolescence. Fortunately, in recent years, researchers have not taken that assumption for granted, and there is now solid evidence that estrogens do indeed organize the brain during puberty, but affect behaviors that might not have been predicted from earlier work in males.

Food guarding is a sexually dimorphic behavior in rats, with males and females displaying different postural strategies for defending their food source (Field, Whishaw, Forgie, & Pellis, 2004). Neonatal or pubertal ovar-iectomy significantly alters the defense strategy to be more "male-like," whereas adult ovariectomy has no effect. Thus, these data suggest that ovarian hormones during the neonatal and/or adolescent periods actively feminize postural strategies for food defense. Another report demonstrates that pubertal exposure to estradiol feminizes ingestive responses to meta-bolic signals in rats (Swithers, McCurley, Hamilton, & Doerflinger, 2008). Treatment with mercaptoacetate, a drug that interferes with fatty acid ox-idation, causes an increase in food intake in male rats but not in females. Ovariectomy in adulthood does not affect this sex difference. However, females that are ovariectomized prior to puberty show a male-like response to mercaptoacetate (i.e., increased food intake), and this effect of prepubertal ovariectomy can be prevented by treatment with estradiol during the time of puberty.

Ovarian hormones may also program mothering during puberty, at least in mice. Maternal behavior in rodents is studied by monitoring mother–pup interactions and quantifying how much time she spends with the pups, espe-cially crouching over them or licking and grooming them, and how quickly she retrieves the pups if they are removed from the nest. If female mice are ovariectomized before puberty and then examined for maternal behavior in adulthood, they spend less time with pups, take longer to retrieve them, and retrieve fewer of them relative to either females that are ovariectomized in adulthood or females that are ovariectomized before puberty *and* given estradiol replacement during the time of puberty (Kercmar, Snoj, Tobet, & Majdic, 2014). If you are wondering how any of these female mice could be mothers if they had been ovariectomized, technically you are right. The mice in this study had not themselves become pregnant or given birth. However, it turns out that mice and rats can't really help themselves if presented with squirming newborns; they seem to be compelled to care for them, even if they can't actually nourish them. So, in this study, foster pups were used to assess the quality and quantity of maternal care. Sure enough, the presence of estradiol during puberty seems to organize the female mouse brain in a way that changes her maternal behavior in adulthood (Kercmar et al., 2014).

As discussed elsewhere in this book, adolescence is the time when rec-reational drug use is most often initiated (see Chapter 8). Although girls and women are less likely than boys and men to use cocaine or other psychostimulants, if they do start down the path of drug use, then they are more vulnerable to abuse and addiction. Animal models point to estradiol as the likely culprit in adulthood. For example, in female rats, estradiol treatment facilitates self-administration of cocaine, increases cocaine intake, and heightens the motivation to seek cocaine; these effects of estradiol are not seen in males (Becker & Hu, 2008). These experiments demonstrate activational effects of estradiol on drug-seeking behavior in adults. Studies also suggest that estradiol, acting during the time of puberty, exerts organizational effects on neural circuits underlying motivation, programming sex differences in vulnerability to drugs of abuse, but not in the way you might think. Perry, Westenbroek, and Becker (2013) looked at self-administration of cocaine in three groups of female rats: ovariectomized prior to puberty with estradiol replacement during the time of puberty, ovariectomized prior to puberty without hormone replacement, and ovariectomized in adulthood (ovaries intact during puberty). After estradiol or vehicle replacement in all groups as adults, the rats were tested for how quickly they would learn to self-administer cocaine and also how hard they would work to obtain cocaine. It turned out that pubertal hormones did not influence acquisition of cocaine self-administration, such that estradiol facilitated acquisition regardless of pubertal hormone status. However, the *motivation* to work for cocaine was affected by pubertal hormone status: The prepubertally ovariectomized rats that received estradiol during puberty gave up faster than the other two groups. In other words, the presence of estradiol during puberty appeared to program a reduced motivation to seek cocaine (Perry et al., 2013). Therefore, in contrast to estradiol being a liability in adulthood in terms of enhancing vulnerability to drug misuse in females, it may actually be an asset during puberty in terms of protecting females against this vulnerability.

Finally, even though we are still playing catch-up in research on females, evidence of organizational effects of gonadal hormones on the neocortex is starting to emerge (Piekarski, Boivin, & Wilbrecht, 2017). In mice, excitatory/inhibitory balance in medial prefrontal cortex shifts right around the onset of puberty toward higher inhibitory tone onto pyramidal projection neurons. Prepubertal ovariectomy prevents this increase in inhibitory tone, but if estradiol and progesterone are replaced at the time of ovariectomy, then the expected increase in inhibitory tone occurs. This effect of ovarian hormones is organizational, not activational, because postpubertal ovariectomy does not affect the inhibitory tone in this area. Moreover, if prepubertal mice are treated with ovarian hormones to mimic an earlier onset of puberty, then maturation of inhibitory tone is advanced. What do these organizational effects in the prefrontal cortex mean for pubertal maturation of executive function? We do not have a clear answer on that just yet. However, it turns out that the developmental shift in excitatory/inhibitory balance is temporally correlated with a developmental shift in performance in a four-choice odor discrimination and reversal task that is dependent on the integrity of prefrontal cortex. In this task, mice first learn that a food reward can be obtained in a cup scented with one odor; in the reversal phase, they must learn that a different odor predicts the cup containing food. Prepubertal mice learn the reversal more readily than postpubertal mice, indicating pubertal maturation is associated with a decrease in behavioral flexibility. Early treatment with estradiol and progesterone produced an adult behavioral phenotype in the reversal learning task, just as it advanced inhibitory maturation (Piekarski et al., 2017). However, mice that are ovariectomized prepubertally and tested postpubertally in the reversal task also show the adult phenotype, so it appears that while ovarian hormones are sufficient to induce a decrease in behavioral flexibility, they are not necessary for its developmental manifestation. Clearly, much remains to be learned about organizational effects of estradiol and progesterone on adult female behaviors. However, from these initial findings in the context of drug seeking and prefrontal function, it is becoming obvious that ovarian hormones can act as mediators of pubertal brain organization.

Hormonal Organization of Behavior, Sex Differences, and Evolution

As the previously discussed studies in males and females indicate, testicular hormones have relatively profound organizational effects on male social behaviors, while ovarian hormones appear to be less influential in organizing female social behaviors. Part of this apparent discrepancy may simply reflect that the bulk of the research to date on organizational effects of pubertal hormones on social behavior has been conducted with male subjects, and if parallel studies were performed in females, we might learn about equally profound effects of ovarian hormones on female social behaviors. However, we think there may be something much more interesting going on, so we'll throw an idea out there in hopes of spawning research to empirically test it. The idea starts with thinking about the whole purpose of puberty and adolescence from an evolutionary perspective, which is to become an adult to procreate and pass on one's genes. To the extent that the biological and behavioral demands of procreation are different in males and females (and this is a pretty big extent for most mammals), then it stands to reason that the selection pressures for what gets organized by hormones during puberty may be very different for males and females. For females, reproductive success is all about having sufficient energy reserves built up to sustain a pregnancy and then, once pregnant, maintaining those reserves and eating for 2 or 3 (or 10) until those pups are weaned. For males, on the other hand, reproductive success is all about having the stuff to outcompete competitors for a potential mate's attention and proving that he can defend his territory. Hence, we posit that evolution has selected for organizational effects of gonadal hormones during puberty that serve to optimize reproductive fitness and that selection pressures are different for females and males. If this is true, then we would also expect that the nitty gritty of what neural circuits and behaviors are organized by gonadal hormones during puberty is going to be a function of both the sex and the species in question.

Clearly there is more work to be done in this area, especially with respect to the role of ovarian hormones in the pubertal organization of brain and behavior, and, if fact, this may be in the cards. The National Institutes of Health (2015) released an official notice that it "expects that sex as a biological variable will be factored into research designs, analyses, and reporting in vertebrate animal and human studies." So stay tuned, as there is undoubtedly more to be revealed concerning how hormones organize and activate the social brain of both males and females throughout adolescence.

Recommended Reading

Baum, M. J. (2009). Sexual differentiation of pheromone processing: links to male-typical behavior and partner preference. *Hormone and Behavior, 55,* 579–588.

Beltz, A. M., & Berenbaum, S. A. (2013). Cognitive effects of variations in pubertal timing: is puberty a period of brain organization for human sex-typed cognition? *Hormone and Behavior, 63,* 823–828.

Juraska, J. M., Sisk, C. L., & DonCarlos, L. L. (2013). Sexual differentiation of the adolescent rodent brain: hormonal influences and developmental mechanisms. *Hormone and Behavior, 64,* 203–210.

7

Stress and the Adolescent Brain

The Perfect Storm

Around the turn of the 20th century, the psychologist G. Stanley Hall published his lengthy two-volume work with the equally lengthy title of *Adolescence: Its Psychology and Its Relation to Physiology, Anthropology, Sociology, Sex, Crime, Religion and Education* (Hall, 1904). With chapters ranging from the stolid "Growth of Parts and Organs During Adolescence," to the sentimental "Adolescent Love," Hall's tome marked the beginning of studying adolescence with the novel angle that this was a rather unique period in an individual's maturation. Although certainly not the major emphasis of *Adolescence* (Arnett, 2006), Hall's book is largely remembered for the suggestion that this stage of development was a time of "storm and stress," when emotional upheaval was commonplace and expected. Most people would agree that adolescence is a life stage associated with significant stress. However, most people would also agree that referring to adolescence as an inevitably stormy, stressful time may be a bit too dramatic. Drama aside, psychologists and neuroscientists are starting to appreciate the role that stress plays in affecting the emotions of adolescents and also how stress and stress-related hormones may actually shape the structure and function of the brain during this period of development (Eiland & Romeo, 2013; Romeo, 2017).

Stress

The word *stress* means different things to different people. In fact, scientists who devote their careers to studying how stress affects the body do not always agree on the same definition of stress (Kagan, 2016; McEwen & McEwen, 2016). For the present discussion, however, we view stress as any internal or external event significant enough to perturb one's homeostasis, with homeostasis referring to the stability of physiological systems within a relatively narrow range to maintain life (e.g., body temperature, glucose levels; Romeo & McEwen, 2006).

Of importance here is that when one experiences a stressor (i.e., the thing knocking us out of homeostasis), whether it be physical, such as an infection or exposure to extreme cold, or psychological, like worry, a cascade of hormones is released to put one's body back in balance. This active physiological process of returning an individual to homeostasis is a process termed *allostasis*. This allostatic hormonal stress response is a double-edged sword, however. In the short term, we need these hormones released during times of stress to help us survive the challenge and bring us back to an even keel. On the other hand, if this hormonal response is chronically engaged or not terminated in a timely fashion, then the prolonged exposure to these hormones can lead to a situation called allostatic load and, in extreme cases, can turn into allostatic overload—when these stress-related hormones become "toxic." Simply put, you can't live without the hormones released during stress, but you also can't live well with too much of them for extended periods of time.

The Hormonal Stress Response

So, what are these stress-related hormones and where do they come from? In response to a stressor, two major physiological systems are activated, responding in parallel, but on slightly different time scales. The first is the sympathetic adrenomedullary (SAM) system, which is activated within milliseconds of encountering a stressor. This system allows for the immediate release of norepinephrine (aka noradrenaline) from neurons of the peripheral sympathetic nervous system and epinephrine (aka adrenaline) from the medulla of the adrenal gland. These chemical transmitters are the "first responders" on the scene and mediate the transient physiological fight-or-flight reactions common in many stressful situations, such as increased heart rate, blood pressure, and respiration (Stratakis & Chrousos, 1995). Although important to our survival during stress, the norepinephrine and epinephrine released into our circulation do not readily cross the blood–brain–barrier (BBB) and thus are not all that germane to our discussion of stress and adolescent neurobiological function (notably, however, these peripherally released hormones can modulate neurotransmitter activity in the brain through indirect pathways, like the vagus nerve (McIntyre, McGaugh, & Williams, 2012).

The second system does directly influence our brain and is called the hypothalamic–pituitary–adrenal (HPA) axis. This system responds on a more protracted time course than the SAM component, taking a couple of minutes to really come up to speed (Herman et al., 2003; Sapolsky, Romero, & Munck, 2000). The HPA response begins when a group of neurons in the hypothalamus, called the paraventricular nucleus (PVN), secretes a hormone into the blood vessels that connect the hypothalamus and anterior pituitary gland. This hormone is corticotrophin-releasing hormone (CRH; aka corticotrophin-releasing factor), and it stimulates the pituitary gland to produce and secrete another hormone, adrenocorticotropic hormone (ACTH). ACTH, in turn, is released into our general circulation and provokes the cortex of the adrenal gland to synthesize and release yet another hormone called cortisol, the business end of the HPA axis. The domino-like process that leads to the eventual release of cortisol is why the full HPA response takes a bit longer to come online compared to the immediate SAM response (Figure 7.1).

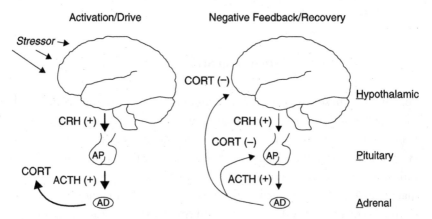

Figure 7.1. The hypothalamic–pituitary–adrenal (HPA) axis. A simplified schematic of the activation of the HPA axis as well as the negative feedback that permits the axis to return to baseline after a stressor has been terminated. AD = adrenal gland; ACTH = adrenocorticotropin hormone; AP = anterior pituitary; CORT = corticosterone; CRH = corticotropin-releasing hormone; (−) = negative feedback; and (+) = positive drive. Note the thickness of the downward and upward pointing arrows are associated with the increased (thicker) drive or decreased (less thick) negative feedback. Reprinted from R. D. Romeo, 2013, The teenage brain: The stress response and the adolescent brain, *Current Directions in Psychological Science, 22,* 140–145. Used with permission from SAGE.

At this point, there is one small detail needing attention before we talk further about the hormonal cascade mediated by the HPA axis. That is, the specific hormone released from the adrenal glands depends on the species in question. For instance, in humans and other primates, the major stress-induced hormone released from the adrenal cortex is cortisol, while in many rodent species, like rats and mice, the major hormone is corticosterone. So throughout this chapter we will be changing between cortisol and corticosterone when discussing research conducted in humans and rodents, respectively, but both hormones have similar mechanisms of action, bind to the same receptors, and have analogous cellular effects.

Cortisol and corticosterone are steroid hormones and, as such, can easily diffuse across the BBB. Therefore, the brain, with its rich supply of blood, can be in intimate contact with these hormones within minutes of exposure to a stressor. These hormones work through two receptors in the brain: the mineralocorticoid receptor (MR) and the glucocorticoid receptor (GR; de Kloet, Vreugdenhil, Oitzl, & Joels, 1998). Similar to the other steroid receptors discussed in the previous chapters, MRs and GRs act as transcription factors, ultimately inducing or repressing gene expression in the cells in which they reside. These receptors are found in relatively high concentrations throughout neural networks that control emotionality and stress reactivity (de Kloet et al., 1998; McEwen, 2005), so not too surprisingly they have been studied not only in the context of HPA function but in mental health and psychopathology as well (de Kloet, Joels, & Holsboer, 2005).

The HPA axis works in a negative feedback loop similar to that described in the context of HPG axis function in Chapter 2. For the HPA axis, the stress-induced increase in cortisol informs the hypothalamus and pituitary gland to reduce the further production and secretion of CRH and ACTH, respectively (Herman et al., 2003; Sapolsky et al., 2000; Figure 7.1). In addition to the hypothalamus, brain regions like the hippocampus and prefrontal cortex also instruct the hypothalamus to limit CRH release when stimulated by cortisol or corticosterone (Herman et al., 2003; Sapolsky et al., 2000). Recall from earlier chapters (see Chapters 2, 4, 5, and 6) the hypothalamus, hippocampus, and frontal cortex all continue to show substantial structural and functional maturation during puberty and adolescence (Giedd, 2004; Gogtay et al., 2004; Juraska & Markham, 2004; Spear, 2000; Yurgelun-Todd, 2007). Thus, shifts in hormonal stress reactivity during the adolescent stage of development might be expected.

Adolescent Development of the Hormonal Stress Response

Significant life transitions are often marked by substantial changes in physiological systems, and the HPA axis is no exception. Specifically, depending on an individual's stage of development, the magnitude and duration of the stress-induced hormonal response can be quite different. During the neonatal period, for instance, stressors that typically elicit a substantial hormonal stress response in adulthood fail to do so in the neonate (Sapolsky & Meaney, 1986). This stress hyporesponsive period has been proposed to protect the developing neonatal brain, and other organ systems, from some of the adverse effects of stress-related hormones (Sapolsky & Meaney, 1986). Aged animals, on the other hand, show heightened or more prolonged hormonal stress responses compared to younger adults (Sapolsky, 1999), and this greater exposure to cortisol and corticosterone has been suggested to contribute to some of the physiological and cognitive dysfunctions associated with the wear-and-tear of aging (Sapolsky, 1999; Sapolsky, Krey, & McEwen, 1985).

Although these changes in HPA responsiveness during neonatal development and aging have garnered considerable research interest (Lupien, McEwen, Gunnar, & Heim, 2009), we know much less about the changes that take place during adolescence. This is surprising for at least two reasons. First, puberty and adolescence are typically marked by significant changes in neuroendocrine function (see Chapter 2). Second, the clinical literature continually indicates a strong relationship between stress exposure during adolescence and the onset or exacerbation of psychological and mood disorders, such as depression, anxiety, and drug use and abuse (Andersen, 2003; Conger & Petersen, 1984; Costello, Mustillo, Erkanli, Keeler, & Angold, 2003; Dahl, 2004; Ge, Natsuaki, Neiderhiser, & Reiss, 2009; Masten, 1987; Patton & Viner, 2007; Spear, 2000). Given that the quantity and quality of stressors change as an individual enters adolescence (Gest, Reed, & Masten, 1999), might there be a direct causal link between these increased stressors and adolescent psychological dysfunction? And, if so, what role do the hormones of the HPA axis play in this association?

Animal studies have started to shed some light on these questions, describing how adolescent maturation affects hormonal stress reactivity and HPA function (McCormick & Mathews, 2007, 2010; McCormick, Mathews, Thomas, & Waters, 2010; Romeo, 2010a, 2010b, 2018; Romeo, Patel, Pham,

& So, 2016). Studies in rats and mice, for instance, have shown that although basal (i.e., resting) and stress-induced ACTH and corticosterone levels are similar in preadolescent and adult animals, they *recover* from stressors differently. That is, once the physical and/or psychological stressor has been terminated, the periadolescent animal's hormonal stress response takes about twice as long as to return to resting levels compared to adults (Romeo, 2018; Figure 7.2). Putting that into a specific timeframe, this difference in recovery would result in periadolescent animals being exposed to corticosterone for 45 to 60 minutes longer than adults, despite animals at both ages experiencing an identical stressor.

It should be noted that not all stressors are created equal. Although most stressors applied to adolescent animals (e.g., foot shock, restraint, hypoxia, cold exposure) lead to this extended hormonal stress response, a systemic stressor, such as an infection, leads to the opposite difference between periadolescent and adult animals. In this instance, when animals are exposed to the endotoxin lipopolysaccharide, the bacterial cell wall of *E. coli* that tricks the immune system into responding like there's a bacterial infection, corticosterone levels of periadolescent animals recover *faster* from this immunological challenge than adults (Goble et al., 2011). This unique observation might be related to the distinctive way in which lipopolysaccharide activates corticosterone production and secretion from the adrenals, which can be independent of both the hypothalamic and pituitary components of the HPA axis (Elenkov, Kovacs, Kiss, Bertok, & Vizi, 1992; Suzuki, Oh, & Nakano, 1986). Despite the different direction of these findings, these data do highlight the bottom line about hormonal stress reactivity and adolescence in rodents: the recovery of the stress-induced HPA response changes rather substantially during adolescent development.

Corresponding to these animal experiments, human studies have also begun to show that the pubertal and adolescent stages of development are associated with alterations in stress-induced HPA reactivity. In fact, the psychiatry journal *Development and Psychopathology* devoted an entire section of a volume to this matter. These studies generally reported increased hormonal stress reactivity during the adolescent period in both boys and girls (Dahl & Gunnar, 2009; Gunnar, Wewerka, Frenn, Long, & Griggs, 2009; Spear, 2009; Stroud et al., 2009). For instance, compared to children, adolescents react with higher and longer cortisol responses to a variety of psychological and social stressors, and the older an adolescent is, the greater

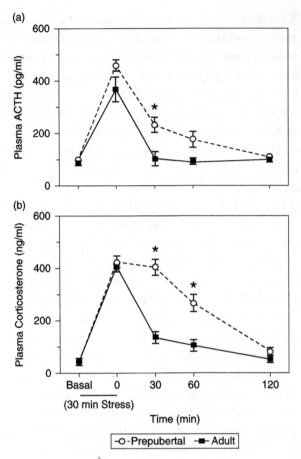

Figure 7.2. Changes in stress-induced hypothalamic–pituitary–adrenal (HPA) reactivity in rats before and after adolescence. Mean (± standard error of the mean) plasma adrenocorticotropic hormone (ACTH; upper panel) and corticosterone (lower panel) concentrations in prepubertal (28 days of age) and adult (77 days of age) male rats in response to 30 minutes of restraint stress (bar beneath x-axis). Asterisks indicate a significant difference between the ages. Reprinted from R. D. Romeo, 2010, Pubertal maturation and programming of hypothalamic–pituitary–adrenal reactivity, *Frontiers in Neuroendocrinology, 31,* 232–240. Used with permission from Elsevier.

their stress-induced hormonal reactivity (Figure 7.3). These data indicate that adolescent-related changes in HPA hormonal stress responses are not limited to laboratory rodents and generally result in greater exposures to adrenal steroids following a variety of stressors.

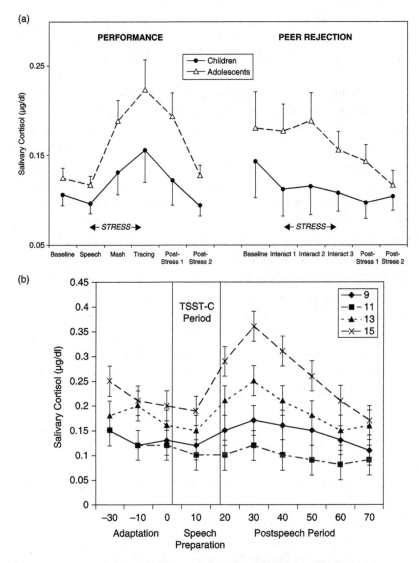

Figure 7.3. Pubertal-related changes in stress-induced hypothalamic–pituitary–adrenal (HPA) reactivity in humans. Mean (± standard error of the mean) salivary cortisol in (A) children (≤12-years-old) and adolescents (≥13-years-old) during performance or peer rejection stress and (B) 9-, 11-, 13-, and 15-year-olds during a Trier Social Stress Test modified for children (TSST-C). Adapted and reprinted from M. R. Gunnar, S. Wewerka, K. Frenn, J. D. Long, & C. Griggs, 2009, Developmental changes in hypothalamus–pituitary–adrenal activity over the transition to adolescence: Normative changes and associations with puberty, *Development and Psychopathology, 21,* 69–85, and L. R. Stroud, E. Foster, G. D. Papandonatos, K. Handwerger, D. A. Granger, K. T. Kivlighan, & R. Niaura, 2009, Stress response and the adolescent transition: Performance versus peer rejection stressors, *Development and Psychopathology, 21,* 47–68. Used with permission from Cambridge University Press.

Stress and the Adolescent Brain

Along with the relatively little we know about how stress reactivity changes during puberty and adolescence, unfortunately, we know even less about what effects these different stress-induced hormonal responses have on the adolescent individual. However, as previously mentioned, the brain regions that continue to show substantial maturation into young adulthood, including the hippocampus and frontal cortex, also have some of the highest levels of GR and MR expression (McEwen, 2005), perhaps making these developing brain areas exquisitely sensitive to stress-related hormones. A growing body of evidence indicates this may indeed be the case.

Because we know so little about the effects of stress on the adolescent brain, we will try to put it into context by first discussing some of the effects that stress has on the structure and function of the adult brain and then comparing that to what we know about stress and the adolescent brain. Specifically, here we will highlight three brain regions that show substantial stress-induced changes in adulthood and also continue to mature during adolescence, namely the hippocampal formation, prefrontal cortex, and amygdala (Giedd & Rapoport, 2010; McEwen, 2012).

Hippocampal Formation

The hippocampal formation is vital to our abilities to remember facts or general knowledge, usually referred to as declarative memory (Squire, 1992). More specifically, the hippocampal formation is imperative in the formation of *new* declarative memories. That is, individuals with damage to their hippocampus often suffer from anterograde amnesia, the inability to form new memories, but not necessarily retrograde amnesia, the inability to retrieve old memories. In addition to its role in declarative memory, the hippocampal formation is also important in helping us form spatial and contextual memories and "cognitive maps." Without a hippocampal formation, it would be difficult to remember how to navigate from one location to the next, for instance (Shapiro, 2001). Given the complex nature of forming new declarative and spatial memories, it is not too surprising that the hippocampal formation itself is quite a complex set of structures. Although the hippocampal formation is composed of many parts, here we will focus on only two of its parts: the hippocampus and dentate gyrus.

The hippocampus is comprised of three layers, the most prominent of which is the pyramidal cell layer. These pyramid-shaped neurons, which give the layer its name, have extensive dendritic branches that emanate from their cell bodies. The dendrites that come from the top (or apex) of the neuron are referred to as the apical dendrites, while those that emerge from the bottom (or base) of the neuron are called the basilar dendrites. Both apical and basilar dendrites are packed with dendritic spines, the primary location for excitatory synapses. The hippocampal pyramidal cell layer is often divided into three zones: cornu ammonis (CA) 1, CA2, and CA3. The demarcation between these zones is not arbitrary, as each zone has different functions, projections, and patterns of gene expression (Lein et al., 2007; Patestas & Gartner, 2006).

Similar to the hippocampus, the dentate gyrus also has three layers, and its most prominent is the granular cell layer. The axons of these granular cells, collectively known as the mossy fibers, are the output of the dentate gyrus and synapse on the dendrites of the CA3 hippocampal pyramidal cells, which, in turn, send their axons to the CA1 cells (Patestas & Gartner, 2006). This dentate-to-CA3-to-CA1 circuit has been posited to play a major role in our abilities to build new memories, not only because of the observation that damage to this circuit leads to profound memory impairments but also because of two additional intriguing phenomena that occur within this circuit.

The first interesting phenomenon is long-term potentiation (LTP). LTP occurs when repetitive stimulation of the CA3 axons results in a long-lasting enhancement of the electrical potentials of the postsynaptic CA1 pyramidal neurons. As the name implies, this potentiation can be rather long term, in that LTP can be observed hours, days, or even weeks after the initial repetitive stimulation of the CA3 axons. Thus, LTP has been proposed to be a putative electrophysiological correlate of learning and memory (Maren & Baudry, 1995). It is important to note that LTP is not exclusive to the hippocampal formation or declarative memory (Chapman, Ramsay, Krezel, & Knevett, 2003). That is, LTP is found in brain areas outside the hippocampus, such as the striatum and amygdala, and the LTP exhibited by these areas appear to be important in the formation of procedural and fear memories, respectively.

The second phenomenon is neurogenesis. If you recall from Chapter 3, neurogenesis is the process by which new neurons are added to the brain, a process that continues throughout the lifespan of an individual. Neurogenesis does not occur evenly throughout the brain, however, but instead appears in a few "hot spots," and one of the hottest spots is the dentate gyrus of the hippocampal formation (Gould, 2007). This has led neuroscientists to suggest that the newly born neurons in this area are involved in the development and/or maintenance of new declarative or spatial memories (Zhao, Deng, & Gage, 2008). Although it is not entirely clear if this suggestion is correct, numerous studies have shown strong correlations between neurogenesis and learning, such that if neurogenesis is blocked or reduced in the dentate gyrus, then hippocampal-dependent learning is compromised (Shors et al., 2001). Now that we have briefly discussed the anatomy and some of the unique properties of the hippocampal formation, let us turn to how stress can affect the structure and function of this critically important brain region.

Stress and the Hippocampal Formation

We all know that stress can influence our abilities to learn and remember information. Less appreciated, however, is how stress-related hormones mediate these changes in our cognitive abilities. Both the pyramidal and granular cell layers of the hippocampal formation are loaded with GR and MR and thus are especially sensitive to cortisol (de Kloet, Oitzl, & Joels, 1999). During times of intense, chronic stress, neurons in these areas start to undergo fundamental changes in their structure and function. One consistent observation in the pyramidal cells of adults is a change in the morphology or shape of these neurons, particularly in the CA3 area, following weeks of intense stress (McEwen, 1999; McEwen & Margarinos, 1997). Specifically, male rats or mice that are exposed to restraint stress intermittently for a few weeks (restraint is a commonly used and potent stressor in laboratory rodents; Buynitsky & Mostofsky, 2009) show significant reductions in the number of apical dendrites found on hippocampal CA3 neurons (Magarinos & McEwen, 1995a; Watanabe, Gould, Cameron, Daniels, & McEwen, 1992; Watanabe, Gould, & McEwen, 1992; Figure 7.4).

This effect appears to be dependent on the stress-induced release of corticosterone, as administering a compound, cyanoketone, which blocks the production of corticosterone, impedes the stress-induced dendritic atrophy of the CA3 pyramidal neurons (Magarinos & McEwen, 1995b). Moreover, one can reproduce these effects of chronic stress on the CA3 neurons by long-term treatment with corticosterone itself (Woolley, Gould, & McEwen, 1990). Although this stress-induced dendritic retraction is most conspicuous in the CA3 region, dendrites of the pyramidal neurons of the CA1 area,

(a)   (b)

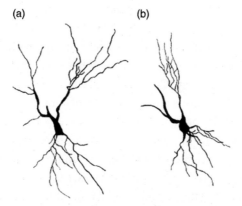

Figure 7.4. Stress and adult hippocampus. Drawings of Golgi-stained hippocampal pyramidal neurons in rats (A) under control conditions or (B) exposed to chronic restraint stress. Adapted and reprinted from Y. Watanabe, E. Gould, H. A. Cameron, D. C. Daniels, & B. S. McEwen, 1992, Phenytoin prevents stress- and corticosterone-induced atrophy of CA3 pyramidal neurons, *Hippocampus, 2,* 431–435. Used with permission from John Wiley and Sons, Inc.

as well granular cells of the dentate gyrus, also demonstrate decreased dendritic complexity in response to chronic stress (Sousa, Lukoyanov, Madeira, Almeida, & Paula-Barbosa, 2000).

Similar to these findings in laboratory animals, human studies using noninvasive neuroimaging techniques, such as magnetic resonance imaging, have demonstrated that individuals reporting high levels of perceived chronic stress show reduced hippocampal volumes (Gianaros et al., 2007). A decrease in hippocampal volume is also observed in patients with Cushing's syndrome, an endocrine disorder marked by high cortisol secretion (i.e., hypercortisolemia; Starkman, Gebarski, Berent, & Schteingart, 1992). Thus, these data suggest that, like the research on experimental animal models, prolonged exposure to cortisol can lead to hippocampal remodeling in humans.

Based on these structural changes in the hippocampal formation, it was predicted that chronic stress would also affect LTP. Indeed, long-term exposure to stress or high levels of corticosterone does significantly reduce LTP (Pavlides, Nivon, & McEwen, 2002). In parallel to these structural and physiological changes, animals exposed to chronic stress demonstrate impaired performance on hippocampal-dependent learning and memory tasks (Conrad, Galea, Kuroda, & McEwen, 1996). For instance, rats exposed to the same stress procedure that reduces CA3 dendritic branching (i.e., 3 weeks of restraint) show poor performance in the Y-maze, an apparatus designed to assess their spatial memory (Conrad et al., 1996).

As if these effects of stress on the structure of pyramidal neurons, LTP, and memory tasks weren't enough, exposure to long periods of stress can also lead to dramatic reductions in neurogenesis. It has been reported that chronic stress can decrease the rates of neurogenesis in the dentate gyrus by about 50% (Dranovsky & Hen, 2006; Gould, McEwen, Tanapat, Galea, & Fuchs, 1997; Pham, Nacher, Hof, & McEwen, 2003). Although these experiments on stress and neurogenesis have only been conducted on laboratory animals and noninvasive methods for measuring neurogenesis in humans are not currently available, it is tempting to speculate that the reduced size of the hippocampal formation in humans experiencing chronic stress, as previously discussed (Gianaros et al., 2007), may be partially mediated by decreases in neurogenesis.

At this point, one may wonder whether if one experiences a period of prolonged stress, are they destined to live the rest of their life with withered hippocampal pyramidal cells and a dentate gyrus bereft of young, newly born neurons? The answer to this question, thankfully, appears to be no. That is, if animals are removed from chronically stressful conditions and allowed to recover in relative peace, then pyramidal cells will begin to rebranch and neurogenesis will ramp back up in as little as 10 days (Conrad, Magarinos, LeDoux, & McEwen, 1999; Heine, Maslam, Zareno, Joels, & Lucassen, 2004). These experiments indicate that stress may disrupt the normal structure and function of the hippocampal formation, but given enough time to recover, the hippocampus can display remarkable elasticity.

The previously mentioned studies clearly show that the adult hippocampal formation is sensitive to stress and stress-related hormones. Less clear is how stressors influence the structure and function of the still developing adolescent hippocampus. Studies have reported that adolescent hippocampal pyramidal neurons show reduced dendritic branching in response to chronic restraint stress, similar to what is seen in adults (Eiland, Ramroop, Hill, Manely, & McEwen, 2012; Figure 7.5). Moreover, one of the earliest studies to assess the effects of chronic stress during adolescence on the structure of the hippocampus showed that chronic variable stress (CVS; e.g., restraint, exposure to cold, loud noises) during puberty resulted in a significantly smaller

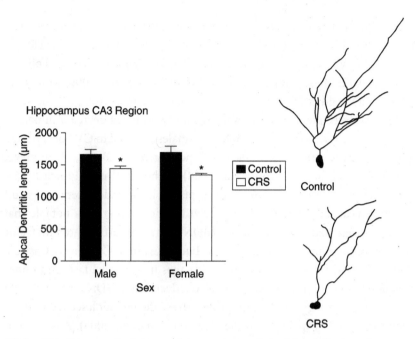

Figure 7.5. Stress and adolescent hippocampus. Apical dendritic length (μm) in the CA3 region of the hippocampus and drawings of Golgi-stained hippocampal pyramidal neurons in male and female adolescent rats under control conditions or those exposed to chronic restraint stress (CRS). Asterisks indicate a significant difference between the experimental conditions. Adapted and reprinted from L. Eiland, J. Ramroop, M. N. Hill, J. Manely, & B. S. McEwen, 2012, Chronic juvenile stress produces corticolimbic dendritic architectural remodeling and modulates emotional behavior in male and female rats, *Psychoneuroendocrinology, 37,* 39–47. Used with permission from Elsevier.

hippocampus in adulthood (Isgor, Kabbaj, Akil, & Watson, 2004). This study also found that these animals exposed to CVS during adolescence showed deficits on learning and memory tasks (Isgor et al., 2004). These structural and behavioral effects were observed 30 days following the termination of the chronic stress exposure during adolescence, suggesting these stress-induced changes last longer (or may take longer to appear) than those seen in adults.

Another way in which the adolescent hippocampal formation responds differentially to stressors than that of adults is in the context of neurogenesis. Remember that adolescence is marked by decreases in neurogenesis (see Chapter 3), such that animals in the earlier stages of adolescence have much higher levels of neurogenesis than animals in the later stages of adolescence or adulthood (Cowen, Takase, Fornal, & Jacobs, 2008; Crews, He, & Hodge, 2007; He & Crews, 2007; Heine et al., 2004; Ho, Villacis, Svirsky, Foilb, & Romeo, 2012; Hodes, Yang, van Kooy, Santollo, & Shors, 2009; Kim et al., 2004; McDonald & Wojtowicz, 2005; Shome, Sultana, Siddiqui, & Romeo, 2018). Interestingly, however, unlike the stress-induced decrease in neurogenesis usually seen in adults, adolescent males exposed to CVS or repeated restraint stress demonstrate *increased* neurogenesis (Barha, Brummelte, Lieblich, & Galea, 2011; Toth et al., 2008). Although it is still unclear why the effects of stress on neurogenesis displayed by the adolescent and adult dentate gyrus are diametrically opposed to one another, it is notable that brain-derived neurotrophic factor (BDNF), an important growth factor in promoting neurogenesis (Sairanen, Lucas, Ernfors, Castren, & Castren, 2005), is regulated by stress at these two ages in a parallel fashion to neurogenesis. That is, chronic stress leads to a decrease in BDNF expression in the adult dentate gyrus, while repeated stress during adolescence leads to increased BDNF expression in the dentate (Toth et al., 2008). Another notable aspect of stress on adolescent hippocampal neurogenesis is that there appears to be a difference in how males and females respond, with adolescent females showing stress-induced decreases in neurogenesis, while adolescent males show increases (Barha et al., 2011).

Together, these studies indicate that stress does affect the structure and function of the adolescent and adult hippocampal formation differently. It also appears that the effects of stress may be longer lasting if they occur during adolescence and are somewhat dependent on the sex of the individual. Clearly, more research and a greater understanding of the impact of stress on the hippocampal formation during adolescent development are warranted. In the interim, however, it is safe to say that prolonged exposure to stress during adolescence can literally shape this intricate brain region in some unique ways.

Stress and the Prefrontal Cortex

Stress not only influences our abilities to learn and remember declarative information, but also profoundly affects our emotions. Stress-induced changes in the prefrontal cortex have been implicated in both these cognitive alterations (Holmes & Wellman, 2009). This brain region is of paramount importance in numerous "executive functions," such as working memory, attention, and emotional control (Holmes & Wellman, 2009; Miller, 2000). Although particularly prominent in the human and nonhuman primate brain (Miller, 2000), the prefrontal cortex does appear to have a homolog in the rodent brain (albeit less complex) loosely called the medial prefrontal cortex (mPFC; Dalley, Cardinal, & Robbins, 2004; Holmes & Wellman, 2009; Uylings, Groenewegen, & Kolb, 2003). This homology has greatly aided our mechanistic understanding of the effects of stress on the prefrontal cortex, especially at the cellular level (Holmes & Wellman, 2009).

In both humans and rodents, this cortical area has six layers, each with specific cell types, functions, and connections (Dalley et al., 2004; Miller, 2000; Uylings et al., 2003). Of relevance to our discussion here, however, are the pyramidal cells of layers II/III. These neurons are similar in morphology to the hippocampal pyramidal cells mentioned earlier, marked by those complex and bushy apical and basilar dendrites. Animal studies have shown that exposure to chronic stress, or repeated corticosterone administration, leads to significant atrophy of the apical dendrites of these layer II/III pyramidal neurons (Holmes & Wellman, 2009; Liston et al., 2006; Radley et al., 2004; Wellman, 2001; Figure 7.6). Moreover, chronic stress results in attenuated LTP induction between the hippocampus and mPFC (Cerqueira, Mailliet, Almeida, Jay, & Sousa, 2007), indicating these structural changes are accompanied by functional changes as well.

These morphological and physiological alterations are paralleled by behavioral changes predicted by a compromised mPFC. Specifically, learning tasks that require an animal to shift attention among various stimuli or use their working memory, abilities dependent on an intact mPFC (Birrell & Brown, 2000), are harder for animals to perform following chronic stress (Cerqueira et al., 2007; Liston et al., 2006). An interesting functional neuroimaging study using medical students as research subjects also showed that 1 month of chronic psychosocial stress (i.e., studying for board exams) disrupted prefrontal function and led to a poor performance on an attentional control task (Liston, McEwen, & Casey, 2009). These data suggest that both lab animals and humans (at least medical students) respond in similar ways to prolonged stressors in the context of prefrontal function, but whether the structural changes in cortical neurons seen following chronic stress in rodents happens in humans is still unknown.

Similar to the elasticity demonstrated by the hippocampus, these stress-induced changes in prefrontal cortex recover back to baseline if given enough

Untreated   Corticosterone

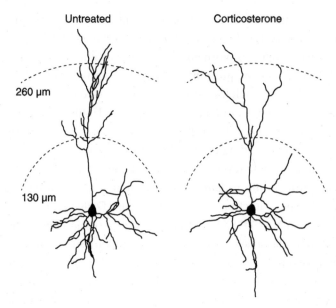

260 µm

130 µm

Figure 7.6. Stress and adult medial prefrontal cortex (mPFC). Drawings of Golgi-stained medial prefrontal cortical neurons of an untreated male rat (left tracing) or one treated with chronic corticosterone (right tracing). Adapted and reprinted from C. L. Wellman, 2001, Dendritic reorganization in pyramidal neurons in medial prefrontal cortex after chronic corticosterone administration. *Journal of Neurobiology, 49,* 245–253. Used with permission from John Wiley and Sons, Inc.

time to recuperate. More specifically, if a previously stressed animal is allowed a 3-week stress-free recovery period, then its mPFC neurons resprout their complex dendrites and appear indistinguishable from those of unstressed, control subjects (Radley et al., 2005). It is presently unclear whether these rats allowed to recover from chronic stress also show improved performance on attention-shifting tasks, but the previously described stressed-out medical students were able to perform their attentional control task as well as the control subjects when tested 1 month after a period of reduced stress (i.e., a vacation; Liston et al., 2009). Thus, chronic stress can significantly affect the structure and function of this key brain area, but luckily, as in the hippocampus, these effects appear to be largely reversible.

This begs the question about whether stress affects the developing adolescent prefrontal cortex, but unfortunately, not much is currently known on this topic. The few animal studies that have been conducted, however, indicate that social (isolation) or psychological (restraint, predator odor) stressors during adolescence can result in long-term changes in markers of synaptic connectivity and reduced dendritic branching in the mPFC (Eiland et al., 2012; Leussis & Andersen, 2008; Leussis, Lawson, Stone, & Andersen, 2008; Wright, Hebert, & Perrot-Sinal, 2008). Leussis and colleagues (Leussis & Andersen, 2008; Leussis et al., 2008) found that isolation stress in adolescent rats leads to decreases in mPFC synaptic proteins (e.g., synaptophysin and spinophilin) that last well into adulthood. It was also found that periadolescent male and female rats exposed to chronic periods of restraint stress displayed reductions in dendritic branching of neurons in the mPFC compared to nonstressed controls (Eiland et al., 2012; Figure 7.7).

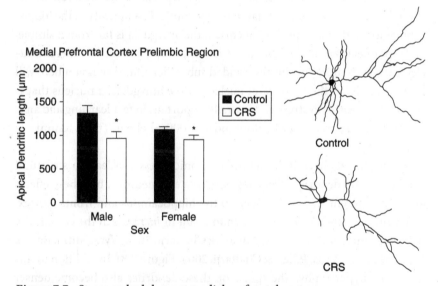

Figure 7.7.   Stress and adolescent medial prefrontal cortex.
Apical dendritic length (μm) in the prelimbic region of the medial prefrontal cortex and drawings of Golgi-stained prefrontal cortical neurons in male and female adolescent rats under control conditions or those exposed to chronic restraint stress (CRS). Asterisks indicate a significant difference between the experimental conditions. Adapted and reprinted from L. Eiland, J. Ramroop, M. N. Hill, J. Manely, & B. S. McEwen, 2012, Chronic juvenile stress produces corticolimbic dendritic architectural remodeling and modulates emotional behavior in male and female rats, *Psychoneuroendocrinology, 37,* 39–47. Used with permission from Elsevier.

The previously discussed studies also found that adolescent stress led to increased fear and depressive-like behaviors in adulthood (Eiland et al., 2012; Leussis & Andersen, 2008; Wright et al., 2008). Although it is difficult to establish whether the stress-induced changes in the adolescent mPFC are responsible for these alterations in adult emotionality, these studies highlight that exposure to stress during adolescence affects the mPFC and these effects may be relatively long lasting, persisting at least into early adulthood.

Stress and the Amygdala

Along with the hippocampal formation and prefrontal cortex, the amygdala has also been reported to be a major target of stress-related hormones. Before we explore what stress does to the amygdala, let us say a few words about the amygdala itself. Similar to the anatomical complexity of the hippocampal formation and prefrontal cortex, the amygdala is far from a simple, homogenous brain region. In fact, it is composed of about 10 different nuclei, each with more specifically divided subnuclei. Our discussion here will center mainly on the basolateral nucleus of the amygdala, a nucleus that is strikingly sensitive to stress and is vitally important in fear learning and anxiety (Fendt & Fanselow, 1999; Roozendaal, 2000; Shekhar, Truitt, Rainnie, & Sajdyk, 2005).

Studies in rats have indicated that chronic stress can lead to structural changes in the dendritic branches of basolateral neurons, but these effects are a bit different from those seen in the hippocampus and frontal cortex. Here, chronic stress has been shown to result in *increases* in the complexity of basolateral dendrites (Vyas, Jadhav, & Chattarji, 2006; Vyas, Mitra, Rao, & Chattarji, 2002; Vyas, Pillai, & Chattarji, 2004; Figure 7.8). In addition to this "dendritic hypertrophy," the spines on these dendrites also become denser (Mitra, Jadhav, McEwen, Vyas, & Chattarji, 2005; Vyas et al., 2006). These effects of stress on the basolateral neurons can be mimicked by treating rats with corticosterone (Mitra & Sapolsky, 2008), indicating the effects of stress on the amygdala are due in part to the stress-induced increase in corticosterone. These changes in the amygdala are also accompanied by significant changes in behaviors influenced by the amygdala. That is, rats exposed to these stressful procedures resulting in dendritic hypertrophy also show significant increases in their anxiety-like behaviors (Conrad et al., 1999; Mitra et al., 2005; Vyas & Chattarji, 2004; Vyas et al., 2002, 2006).

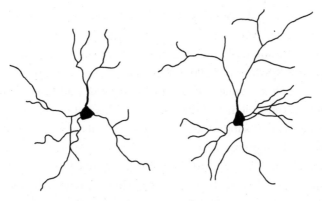

Figure 7.8. Stress and adult amygdala. Drawings of Golgi-stained neurons from the basolateral nucleus of the amygdala in rats under control conditions (left tracing) or prolonged immobilization stress (right trace). Adapted and reprinted from A. Vyas, R. Mitra, B. S. S. Rao, & S. Chattarji, 2002, Chronic stress induces contrasting patterns of dendritic remodeling in hippocampus and amygdala neurons, *Journal of Neuroscience, 22,* 6810–6818. Used with permission from Society for Neuroscience.

Because the effects of stress on the morphology of neurons in the hippocampal formation and prefrontal cortex are reversible, additional studies were conducted to assess whether the stress-induced increase in the dendritic complexity of neurons in the amygdala were temporary or enduring. It was found that even when animals were given 21 stress-free days of recovery they continued to show increased dendritic branching (Vyas et al., 2004). Remember that 3 weeks of recovery is a sufficient amount of time for hippocampal and prefrontal cells to return to their prestress shape. Thus, it appears that stress-induced changes in the structure of the neurons in the basolateral amygdala are longer lasting compared to the morphological changes caused by stress in the either the hippocampal formation or prefrontal cortex.

Similar to the lack of data regarding the effects of stress on the adolescent hippocampus and cortex, we know virtually nothing about how stress affects the structure of the adolescent amygdala in general or the basolateral nucleus specifically. However, a study in rats showed that a few days of restraint stress and foot shocks during adolescence can result in long-term changes in both fearfulness and markers of synaptic plasticity in the amygdala (Tsoory, Guterman, & Richter-Levin, 2009). In particular, it was found that animals that experienced juvenile stress displayed greater fear learning

in adulthood, as well as increased expression of neural cell adhesion molecule L1 in the basolateral nucleus of the amygdala (Tsoory et al., 2009). As
neural cell adhesion molecule L1 is involved in neural maturation and plasticity (Maness & Schachner, 2007), these data suggest that stress experienced
during the adolescent stage of developmental can lead to later changes in
the structure and function of the amygdala. This notion has received additional experimental support as adolescent animals exposed to chronic restraint stress do show an increase in the dendritic branching of neurons in
the basolateral nucleus (Eiland et al., 2012; Figure 7.9). However, it is currently unknown whether these structural changes return to baseline levels
following a break from stress. Clearly, further research is required in this area
to establish whether the effects of stress on the adolescent amygdala are similar to or different from those effects observed in adults and, importantly,

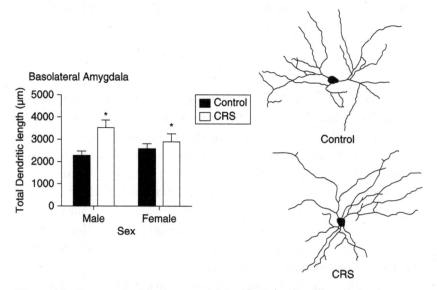

Figure 7.9. Stress and adolescent amygdala. Total dendritic length (μm)
in the basolateral nucleus of the amygdala and drawings of Golgi-stained
amygdalar neurons in male and female adolescent rats under control conditions
or those exposed to chronic restraint stress (CRS). Asterisks indicate a
significant difference between the experimental conditions. Adapted and
reprinted from L. Eiland, J. Ramroop, M. N. Hill, J. Manely, & B. S. McEwen,
2012, Chronic juvenile stress produces corticolimbic dendritic architectural
remodeling and modulates emotional behavior in male and female rats,
Psychoneuroendocrinology, 37, 39–47. Used with permission from Elsevier.

whether any stress-induced changes in the adolescent amygdala contribute to the reported increases in anxiety disorders following a stressful adolescence (Grant et al., 2003; Turner & Lloyd, 2004).

The Perfect Storm?

The previous three sections have highlighted some of what we know regarding stress and the adolescent brain. Although the data are slim relative to what we know in adults, it appears that the adolescent brain is indeed affected by stressors and these effects are sometimes different from what we see in adults. It also appears from the previously reviewed studies that the effects of stress on the adolescent brain may be longer lasting, and perhaps even permanent, when compared to adults. This leads to the question: Is the storm and stress of adolescence, coupled with the continued maturation of the adolescent brain, creating a perfect storm for stress-related vulnerabilities to occur? This is, after all, the time in one's life marked by a major uptick in stress-related psychological disorders (Lee, Heimer et al., 2014), with one in five adolescents afflicted by a serious psychological or mental health issue (Kessler et al., 2005), so something must account for this significant change.

In keeping with this weather metaphor, let us consider the various "fronts" that we have alluded to in this chapter and their possible convergence to create such a storm. First, as previously mentioned, the quality and quantity of stressors change during adolescence (Arnett, 1999; Gest et al., 1999), such that, relative to childhood, stressors are often more frequent during this stage of life and take on novel forms, such as increased tensions with caregivers and peers, complex intimate relationships, and entering the workforce. Second, as previously presented, hormonal stress reactivity increases during the adolescent period, typically showing greater or more protracted stress responses (Dahl & Gunnar, 2009; McCormick & Mathews, 2007; Romeo, 2010a, 2010b; Romeo et al., 2016; Spear, 2009). Third, areas of the brain that continue to mature during adolescence, such as the hippocampus, prefrontal cortex, and amygdala (see Chapters 4 and 5), are exquisitely sensitive to stress-related hormones (McEwen, 2005). Thus, the intersection of these factors could lead to a unique and significant set of negative outcomes on the short- and long-term function of the adolescent brain. It is important to note, however, despite a lot of correlative data to support the notion that chronic stress exposure during adolescence can lead to psychological dysfunctions in adulthood (Grant, Compas, Thurm, McMahon, & Gipson, 2004; Grant et al., 2003; Turner & Lloyd, 2004), empirical support for this "perfect storm" assertion is currently lacking (Eiland & Romeo, 2013).

A Harbor in the Tempest

The previously outlined idea indicates that the dramatic changes in stress reactivity coupled with the continued maturation of the brain might make the adolescent individual extremely susceptible to stress-related neurobiological perturbations. However, these significant transitions may also afford an important opportunity to intervene and combat these perturbations. Put another way, if parts of the adolescent brain are malleable, thus making them especially prone to stress, then wouldn't this pliability allow for the opportunity to intervene and counter these insults?

A number of provocative studies using environmental enrichment indicate that adolescence may indeed be a stage of development that might reap the benefits of exposure to stimulating, complex surroundings. In these studies, enrichment usually means that animals are living in larger cages than usual, with toys, numerous cage mates, and access to a running wheel, or some other form of voluntary exercise (Fox, Merali, & Harrison, 2006; Mora, Segovia, & del Arco, 2007). These experiments show that earlier troubles caused by prenatal or neonatal stress can largely be mitigated by utilizing environmental enrichment during adolescence (Bredy, Humpartzoomian, Cain, & Meaney, 2003; Bredy, Zhang, Grant, Diorio, & Meaney, 2004; Francis, Diorio, Plotsky, & Meaney, 2002; Morley-Fletcher, Rea, Maccari, & Laviola, 2003). For instance, the heightened stress reactivity typically displayed by prenatally stressed offspring in adulthood is normalized if the animals are raised in an enriching environment during adolescence (Morley-Fletcher et al., 2003; Figure 7.10). Along these lines, children that experience more than their fair share of stressful life events appear to be protected from developing depression during adolescence if these children, and their parents, report a greater level of closeness and social enrichment (Ge et al., 2009).

In conclusion, the research described in this chapter present some of the unique ways in which adolescents respond to stressors and how their stress responses may affect their brains in relatively idiosyncratic ways. These studies also provide hope for the unlucky individuals who do happen to experience significant amounts of stress for prolonged periods before or during

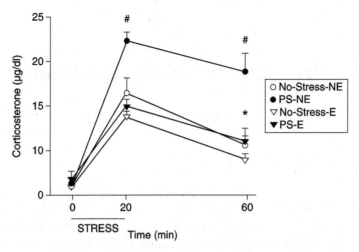

Figure 7.10. Environmental enrichment during adolescence mitigating prenatal stress. Restraint stress-induced plasma corticosterone response in adolescent male rats that were prenatally stressed or not (PS and No-stress, respectively) and then exposed to nonenriched environmental conditions (NE) or enriched environmental conditions during adolescence. Reprinted from S. Morley-Fletcher, M. Rea, S. Maccari, & G. Laviola, 2003, Environmental enrichment during adolescence reverses the effects of prenatal stress on play behaviour and HPA axis reactivity in rats, *European Journal of Neuroscience, 18,* 3367–3374. Used with permission from John Wiley and Sons, Inc.

adolescence. Although it is certainly easier said than done, it appears that timely interventions, along with social support, may not only pay dividends in the short term during a stressful adolescence, but may also offer lasting benefits for an individual's mental health and neurobiological function into young adulthood, and possibly beyond.

Recommended Reading

Fuhrmann, D., Knoll, L. J., & Blakemore, S-J. (2015). Adolescence as a sensitive period of brain development. *Trends in Cognitive Sciences, 19,* 558–566.

McEwen, B. S., & Lasley, E. N. (2002). *The end of stress as we know it.* New York, NY: Dana Press.

Sapolsky, R. M. (2004). *Why zebras don't get ulcers* (3rd ed.). New York, NY: Henry Holt.

8

Drugs and the Adolescent Brain

Eggs Anyone?

The TV public service announcement (PSA) is iconic: a hot frying pan with butter on the stove top, the cracking of an egg, followed by an intense sizzle, all with the voiceover: "This is drugs. This is your brain on drugs. Any questions?" The brain figures predominantly in any discussion of drug use and abuse because of its major role in mediating the psychological and behavioral aspects of addiction. However, as the PSA dramatically highlights, it also grabs attention because of the adverse impact of drugs "frying" the brain, with many short- and long-term consequences on its structure and function. Although it has long been recognized that adolescence is a particularly intense time of drug experimentation, increasing attention is being paid to how drugs and the developing adolescent brain interact, sometimes in particularly adverse ways, sparking numerous lines of human and nonhuman animal research. This chapter will highlight some of the ways in which drugs can influence the adolescent brain and its development. Importantly, we will focus on more than just the "usual suspects" of drugs of abuse such as alcohol, nicotine, and marijuana. Specifically, we will also discuss other psychoactive substances widely used by adolescents such as anabolic steroids and commonly prescribed drugs. Although the fried egg metaphor is overdoing it a bit, it is becoming quite clear that drugs can and do influence the adolescent brain in many integral and profound ways (Bava & Tapert, 2010; Witt, 2010).

Adolescence as a Vulnerable Period to Drugs of Abuse

Drug abuse among adolescents is a clear public health concern, and the statistics are staggering. In 2016, the annual Monitoring the Future Study, funded by the National Institutes of Drug Abuse and compiled by researchers at the University of Michigan, indicated that the annual prevalence of use of illicit drugs (e.g., marijuana, hallucinogens, cocaine) in 8th graders is 12%, jumping to 38% by 12th grade. Alcohol usage is particularly striking; its annual prevalence rates are 17% and 56% among 8th and 12th graders, respectively. Although this drug use during adolescence is typically in the context of "experimentation" and not necessarily one of abuse per se (Young et al., 2002), one of the best predictors of developing a problem with substance *abuse* in adulthood is substance *use* during adolescence (Grant & Dawson, 1997; Palmer et al., 2009). For instance, findings in animals showed that repeated alcohol use by adolescent rats predicted greater alcohol use in these same rats as adults (Alaux-Cantin et al., 2013; Pascual, Boix, Felipo, & Guerri, 2009). The reasons for this uptick in drug use during adolescence are not entirely clear but likely happens in part due to changes in the neural systems that mediate reward (Doremus-Fitzwater, Varlinskaya, & Spear, 2010). For instance, as presented earlier in Chapter 5, both human and animal studies indicate significant changes in brain areas that participate in reward and decision-making during the adolescent stage of development (Doremus-Fitzwater et al., 2010; Galvan, 2010). Moreover, monoaminergic neurotransmitter systems that underlie motivation and reward-seeking, particularly the dopaminergic system, show maturational changes in activity and reactivity during adolescence (Murrin, Sanders, & Byland, 2007; Wahlstrom, White, & Luciana, 2010).

In addition to these shifts in motivation, other interesting aspects of drug use in adolescents are their particular sensitivities and physiological and psychological responses they have to drugs. That is, adolescent individuals may experience more of the positive effects of drugs, while experiencing far fewer of the negative effects. This "accentuate the positive, eliminate the negative" phenomenon is particularly apparent in the context of alcohol use. For example, following a hefty dose of alcohol, adolescent rats show greater levels of social behavior (Varlinskaya & Spear, 2002) and less impaired motor coordination (Novier, Diaz-Granados, & Matthews, 2015; White et al., 2002) compared to adults. Adolescent animals also exhibit decreased sensitivity to alcohol's sedative properties compared to adults (Novier et al., 2015; Silveri & Spear, 1998). On the other hand, the physiological and psychological components of the "hangover" after an alcohol binge may be less in adolescent individuals, as studies indicate that adolescent rats show less anxiousness than adults a day after an acute, intense exposure to alcohol (Doremus, Brunell, Varlinskaya, & Spear, 2003).

Taken together, the changes in sensitivity to drugs as well as the changes in reward-related neural circuitry likely contribute to the increase in drug use during adolescence. However, instead of further exploring the myriad mechanisms that lead to increases in adolescence drug use, ably reviewed previously (Doremus-Fitzwater & Spear, 2016; Doremus-Fitzwater et al., 2010; Spear & Varlinskaya, 2010), the rest of this chapter will focus on the consequences of drug exposure on adolescent brain remodeling and development.

"Traditional" Drugs of Abuse: Shaping the Adolescent Brain Under the Influence of Alcohol, Nicotine, and Marijuana

Alcohol

As previously mentioned, the incidence of alcohol use can be quite high among teenagers (Johnston, O'Malley, Bachman, & Schulenberg, 2008). For instance, a survey of secondary school students in New York State indicated that 71% of students are drinkers, while 13% of these are heavy drinkers (i.e., consuming five or more drinks weekly). Although this has many important implications for the increased risk-taking and poor decision-making often engaged in during adolescence (see Chapter 5), alcohol can interfere with the progressive and regressive events associated with brain development that we covered in Chapter 3. To make matters worse, the adolescent brain appears to be particularly sensitive to the neurotoxic effects of alcohol. For instance, when adolescent and adult animals are administered a similar amount of alcohol, the adolescent animals show much more neural damage than the adults (Crews, Braun, Hoplight, Switzer, & Knapp, 2000). One only need to think about the devastating effects that prenatal alcohol exposure can have on the developing brain (Guerri, 2002; Roebuck, Mattson, & Riley, 1998), and the ensuing cognitive dysfunctions in individuals suffering from fetal alcohol syndrome (Mattson & Riley, 1998), to imagine the damage alcohol can do when the adolescent brain is undergoing its remodeling project.

During development, cell proliferation and differentiation play a major role in shaping the ultimate structure and function of the adult brain. As you may recall from Chapters 3 and 7, hippocampal neurogenesis changes during adolescent development (Crews, He, & Hodge, 2007; He & Crews,

2007; Ho, Villacis, Svirsky, Foilb, & Romeo, 2012; Kim et al., 2004). In an effort to determine whether alcohol has any effect on hippocampal neurogenesis during adolescence, researchers gave adolescent rats a single dose of alcohol that resulted in a blood alcohol concentration of about 0.13% (Crews, Mdzinarishvili, Kim, He, & Nixon, 2006). To put this in context, in the United States, the legal driving limit is 0.08%, while an individual with a blood alcohol concentration of 0.35% would be in a drunken stupor and likely unconscious. Thus, although tipsy, these rats would be far from "wasted." The important point to make here, however, is that under these physiologically relevant conditions, cell proliferation in the dentate gyrus was reduced by up to 75% in these alcohol-exposed adolescent rats (Crews et al., 2006). Moreover, when animals were assessed 28 days later, the survival of the cells born during this experimenter-induced bender was diminished by a third. It is important to note that adult rats treated with the same dose of alcohol do show decreases in hippocampal cell proliferation, but these decreases are not as dramatic as those exhibited by the adolescent animals (Crews et al., 2006). Other studies in adolescent male rats found similar results when animals were exposed to alcohol for longer periods of time (a few days to a few weeks), with alcohol-exposed rats during adolescence showing both short- and long-term reductions in hippocampal cell proliferation and neurogenesis (Broadwater, Liu, Crews, & Spear, 2014; Jang et al., 2002; Morris, Eaves, Smith, & Nixon, 2010). On the flip side of cell birth, cell death was noted to be higher in adolescent animals exposed to alcohol compared to controls (Broadwater et al., 2014; Jang et al., 2002), an effect shown to be greater when the exposure to the same amount of alcohol happened during adolescence compared to adulthood (Broadwater et al., 2014). Therefore, these data show that brief or chronic exposure to alcohol can significantly affect cell proliferation, differentiation, and cell death in the adolescent hippocampus and that these effects are more pronounced in the adolescent compared to the adult brain.

Although this may be troubling news for rodents, does alcohol use by adolescent primates, such as humans, lead to similar effects on neurogenesis in the developing dentate gyrus? Unfortunately, due to our current inability to measure neurogenesis in vivo in humans, not to mention the ethical issues inherent in alcohol research in teens, this question has not yet been addressed. An experiment in nonhuman primates, however, has shown that adolescent rhesus monkeys that were allowed to drink ethanol demonstrated diminished hippocampal neurogenesis compared to their sober counterparts (Taffe et al., 2010). Moreover, the ethanol-exposed monkeys had higher levels of cell death in the dentate gyrus, even months after they stopped drinking (Taffe et al., 2010). Together, the data derived from both the rodent and nonhuman primate studies indicate that the developing hippocampal formation can be significantly affected by ethanol consumption, with possible long-term consequences for its neurogenic capacity and functioning. Given alcohol's inhibiting effect on neurogenesis, these data may help explain why the volume of the hippocampus is significantly smaller in adolescent boys and girls diagnosed with alcohol use disorder and dependence compared to their healthy, nonalcohol-dependent teen counterparts (De Bellis et al., 2000).

Although alcohol exposure can clearly affect the wholesale addition (and subtraction) of new neurons, what about the role of alcohol on neuronal connectivity and synaptic plasticity in the adolescent brain? That is, are synapses in the adolescent brain also affected following alcohol use, and can neurons still communicate effectively with one another under the influence? In the adult brain, alcohol can lead to extensive remodeling of dendrites and dendritic spines, particularly in cortical and subcortical regions (Chandler, 2003; Fiala, Spacek, & Harris, 2002; Jones, 1988). More specifically, over the years, a substantial literature has accumulated indicating that adult rodents chronically treated with ethanol show fewer dendrites and dendritic spines in brain areas such as the cerebellum (Tavares, Paula-Barbosa, & Gray, 1983), hippocampal formation (McCullen, Saint-Cyr, & Carlen, 1984; Riley & Walker, 1978), nucleus accumbens (Zhou et al., 2007), and the prefrontal cortex (Cadete-Leite, Alves, Paula-Barbosa, Uylings, & Tavares, 1990). Not surprisingly, these structural alterations are paralleled by functional changes, such as compromised long-term potentiation and cognitive deficits (Blizter, Gil, & Landau, 1990; Ryback, 1973). Although this paragraph has clearly oversimplified an enormous body of research, glossing over many important details and exceptions, the broad conclusion drawn for the literature on chronic alcohol exposure and the adult brain is this: Chronically imbibing large amounts of alcohol generally leads to a poorly functioning adult brain.

Unfortunately, we know relatively little about the impact of alcohol on adolescent brain morphology (Witt, 2010), particularly in the context of the size and shape of the neurons and the structural processes that grow from them. We do know, however, that synaptic activity in the adolescent brain is greatly affected by alcohol, specifically within the hippocampus (White & Swartzwelder, 2004). For instance, using electrophysiological techniques, researchers have shown that ethanol-exposed hippocampal brain slices taken from prepubertal animals display less excitatory electrical activity than ethanol-exposed hippocampal slices taken from adults (Pyapali, Turner, Wilson, & Swartzwelder, 1999; Swartzwelder, Wilson, & Tayyeb, 1995). Although it is unclear what accounts for this pubertal difference in hippocampal excitability, studies have also shown that prepubertal alcohol exposure leads to a greater reduction in an integral part of the N-methyl-D-aspartate receptor, a receptor important in learning and memory and in the actions of the excitatory neurotransmitter glutamate (Pian, Criado, Milner, & Ehlers, 2010). In line with these physiological and biochemical findings, adolescent animals appear to have more trouble learning their way around a maze, a task dependent on a finely tuned hippocampus, when under the influence of alcohol than similarly intoxicated adults (Markwiese, Acheson, Levin, Wilson, & Swartzwelder, 1998), although there is some disagreement whether this holds for all aspects of learning (Chin, Van Skike, & Matthews, 2010).

It is important to note that the hippocampus is not the only place in the brain that shows these differential sensitivities to alcohol before and after adolescent development. In fact, the same research group that discovered that the electrophysiological properties of the prepubertal hippocampus were especially sensitive to the inhibitory effects of alcohol also showed that the adolescent cingulate cortex displays less activity following alcohol exposure compared to adults (Li, Wilson, & Swartzwelder, 2002). As the cingulate cortex is vitally important in helping us make sound judgments and pay attention to our surroundings (Vogt, Finch, & Olson, 1992), it is not too surprising this area is disrupted under the influence of alcohol. These differential age effects of alcohol on the cingulate cortex may also help explain the anecdotal reports of some of the particularly bad decisions made by intoxicated adolescents.

Although alcohol can clearly lead to some negative effects on adolescent brain function in the short term, it also appears that alcohol exposure during adolescence can lead to greater dysfunctions when these same individuals drink later in adulthood. For example, studies in both humans and rodents indicate that prior bouts of bingeing on alcohol can lead to poorer performance on memory tasks when tested later under the acute influence of alcohol in adulthood (Weissenborn & Duka, 2003; White, Ghia, Levin, & Swartzwelder, 2000). Taken together, therefore, this ever-expanding area of research on alcohol and the developing adolescent brain suggests that the hangover a teenager experiences after a heavy night of drinking may last longer than just the headache the next morning.

Nicotine

Similar to the shocking statistics on alcohol consumption during adolescence, tobacco use among teenagers is relatively prevalent. Although the numbers are not as high as those reported for alcohol use, approximately 9% of teenagers (12–17 years of age) indicate that they have used a tobacco product (e.g., cigarettes, cigars, smokeless tobacco) in the last month, with 1.6% reporting daily use (Kasza et al., 2017). As one of the greatest predictors of tobacco consumption in adulthood is tobacco consumption in adolescence (Substance Abuse and Mental Health Services Adminstration, 2009), this does not bode well for the future of teenagers experimenting with tobacco in middle and high school. Although tobacco has clear devastating effects on one's overall health and remains the single most preventable cause of death (Benowitz, 2010), we are just beginning to appreciate the effects that specific chemicals in tobacco, particularly nicotine, have on the structure and function of the adolescent brain.

Upon inhaling cigarette smoke, nicotine rapidly enters the brain when absorbed into the blood through the lungs (or adsorbed through the skin in the case of chewing tobacco). Like research on alcohol, a fair number of studies have attempted to examine why our brains start to crave nicotine once we have had a few experiences with tobacco (Benowitz, 2010). However, of importance here is what type of effects nicotine may have on the remodeling of the adolescent brain.

There is growing evidence that nicotine does indeed affect adolescent and adult individuals differently. If we go back to the lopsided alcohol scenario of "accentuate the positive, eliminate the negative," it appears that adolescent animals also experience greater "positive" effects (i.e., greater reward) and less "negative" effects (i.e., fewer withdrawal effects) of nicotine than adults (O'Dell, 2009). For instance, adolescent rodents show a conditioned place preference to a lower dose of nicotine than adults (Shram & Le, 2010; Vastola, Douglas, Varlinskaya, & Spear, 2002), suggesting that nicotine may be more rewarding in animals prior to puberty. Moreover, prepubertal rats given injections of nicotine show greater behavioral activity and engage in more social behaviors compared to adults (Cao et al., 2010; Trezza, Baarendse, &

Vanderschuren, 2009; Vastola et al., 2002). On the other hand, adolescent animals show less conditioned place and taste aversion (O'Dell, 2009; Shram, Funk, Li, & Le, 2006; Wilmouth & Spear, 2004), as well as reduced hormonal stress responses (Cao et al., 2010), following nicotine exposure compared to similarly treated adults. Intertwined in this differential sensitivity to nicotine before and after puberty, there also appears to be some differences between the sexes in that, given the chance, adolescent female rats will self-administer nicotine at a higher level than adolescent males (Lynch, 2009). Although it is presently unclear what mediates these age- and sex-dependent changes in nicotine sensitivity, it is clear that nicotine has differential effects on the adolescent and adult brain.

Given the shifts in reward value of nicotine in adolescent animals, a number of studies have looked at how nicotine affects the neurons within the nucleus accumbens, a major player in the limbic reward circuit. Studies have found that adolescent rats chronically exposed to nicotine had more elaborate dendritic branching patterns of accumbal neurons than rats that had abstained during adolescence (McDonald et al., 2005). Moreover, this enhanced nicotine-induced dendritic branching appears to be specific to the adolescent stage, as animals treated with chronic nicotine during adulthood did not show these more structurally complex neurons in the accumbens (McDonald et al., 2007). Although it is difficult to establish direct cause-and-effect relationships between specific structural alterations of neurons and behavior, is it possible that the greater rewarding properties of nicotine during adolescence are related to nicotine's ability to tweak these accumbal neurons (Figure 8.1).

In addition to the apparent neuronal growth-promoting effects of nicotine on the adolescent brain, there are plenty of examples in the scientific literature that indicate nicotine can also act as a neurotoxin during this development stage. Specifically, animals administered nicotine throughout the adolescent period of development showed reductions in both neural density and neural projections in the cerebral cortex (Abreu-Villaca, Seidler, Tate, & Slotkin, 2003). These effects were noticeable up to a month following the exposure, even though the doses of nicotine used in this study only resulted in plasma nicotine levels near, or even below, those typically found in regular smokers (Abreu-Villaca et al., 2003).

Human studies have shown that adolescent smokers do not perform as well in cognitive tests and memory tasks compared to their nonsmoking counterparts (Jacobsen et al., 2005). Along these lines, animal experiments

(a)   (b)

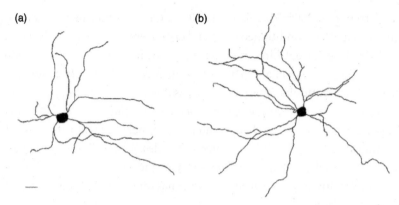

Figure 8.1. Nicotine and morphology of neurons in the adolescent accumbens.
The morphology of neurons in the adolescent nucleus accumbens in rats
exposed to control (left tracing) or nicotine conditions (right tracing). Scale
bar = 20 μm. Reprinted from C. G. McDonald, V. K. Dailey, H. C. Bergstrom,
T. L. Wheeler, A. K. Eppolito, L. N. Smith, & R. F. Smith, 2005, Periadolescent
nicotine administration produces enduring changes in dendritic morphology
of medium spiny neurons from nucleus accumbens, *Neuroscience Letters, 385,*
163–167. Used with permission from Elsevier.

have also found that nicotine can be particularly toxic to the hippocampus.
For instance, mice given prolonged nicotine exposure during adolescence
show greater neuronal and glial apoptosis compared to their nonexposed
controls (Jang et al., 2002; Oliveira-da-Silva et al., 2009) as well as reduced
cell proliferation (Jang et al., 2002). A series of follow-up studies, however,
indicated this increase in hippocampal cell death was relatively brief, in that,
given 5 days to recover, their neuronal and glial cell densities revert back to
normal levels (Oliveira-da-Silva, Manhaes, Cristina-Rodrigues, Filgueiras,
& Abreu-Villaca, 2010). Thus, perhaps there is a silver lining in this smoke
cloud for those teenagers that kick the habit.

It is important to note that not all nicotine-induced changes in the
adolescent brain are structural. For instance, both adolescent and adult
animals exposed to nicotine show significant changes in gene expression in the ventral tegmental area (VTA), a dopamine-rich region of
the brain involved in addiction. What is particularly fascinating about
this discovery is that the specific genes that are influenced by nicotine
at these two stages are quite different. In fact, only 4% of the genes that
are modulated by nicotine are modulated similarly in the adolescent and

adult VTA (Doura, Luu, Lee, & Perry, 2010), while the rest of the genes that are upregulated or downregulated are dependent on the animal's developmental stage.

Along with these particular nicotine-induced changes in the adolescent brain, an emerging area of research has begun to show that nicotine exposure during adolescence can lead to long-term changes in one's emotionality. Specifically, a number of studies have reported that animals given nicotine during adolescence present with higher levels of depressive- and anxiety-like behaviors upon reaching adulthood than adults that were nicotine-free during adolescence (Iniguez et al., 2009; Slawecki, Gilder, Roth, & Ehlers, 2003).

Taken together, it appears the effects of nicotine on the adolescent brain are both widespread and, compared to adults, relatively unique. From tweaking the dendrites of accumbal neurons to modulating one's future emotionality, it is clear that we should not underestimate the impact of nicotine (and other chemicals found in tobacco) on the developing adolescent brain. In fact, secondhand smoke studies have even shown exposure to just tobacco smoke itself can reduce hippocampal neurogenesis (Bruijnzeel et al., 2011; Figure 8.2) and increase anxiety-like behavior in adolescent rats (de la Pena et al., 2016). Perhaps some additions to the warning labels on tobacco products are in order?

Marijuana

Outside of alcohol and tobacco, marijuana (aka cannabis) is one of most commonly used drugs by teenagers (Johnston et al., 2008), with reports indicating that 6% of 12th graders use this illicit drug daily (Jacobus, Bava, Cohen-Zion, Mahmood, & Tapert, 2009; Johnston et al., 2008). These numbers are made more unsettling by the claim that cannabis use during adolescence appears to be a risk factor for the later development of psychotic disorders, such as schizophrenia (Andreasson, Allebeck, Engstrom, & Rydberg, 1987; Arsenault et al., 2002; Casadio, Fernandes, Murray, & Di Forti, 2011; Malone, Hill, & Rubin, 2010; Renard, Krebs, Le Pen, & Jay, 2014). Thus, it is imperative we begin to understand the short- and long-term consequences of cannabis consumption during adolescence, particularly in regards to the developing brain.

The psychoactive ingredient in marijuana is Δ^9-tetrahydrocannabinol, usually abbreviated (thankfully) to THC (Gaoni & Mechoulam, 1964;

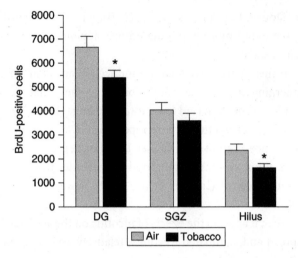

Figure 8.2. Tobacco smoke and cell proliferation in the adolescent dentate gyrus. The number of BrdU-positive cells in sub-regions of the adolescent dentate gyrus following exposure to tobacco smoke (black bars) or room air (grey bars). Reprinted from A. W. Bruijnzeel, R. M. Bauzo, V. Munikoti, G. B. Rodrick, H. Yamada, C. A. Fornal, . . . B. L. Jacobs, 2011, Tobacco smoke diminishes neurogenesis and promotes gliogenesis in the dentate gyrus of adolescent rats, *Brain Research, 1413,* 32–42. Used with permission from Elsevier.

Mechoulam, 1970). THC binds to receptors in the brain called cannabinoid receptors, which are found in the basal ganglia, cortex, and hippocampus (Herkenham et al., 1989, 1991; Pazos, Nunez, Bentio, Tolon, & Romero, 2005). Although the social and neurobiological factors that may mediate the increase in cannabis use during adolescence remain unclear, it appears that adolescent animals respond with less aversion to THC than adults (Schramm-Sapyta et al., 2007). For instance, adult rats show a conditioned place aversion to the environment in which they had previously received repeated THC injections, while adolescent rats do not (Quinn et al., 2008). Thus, similar to the studies that have demonstrated differential reactivity to the rewarding and aversive properties of alcohol and nicotine (O'Dell, 2009; Silveri & Spear, 1998), the relative lack of negative reactions to THC prior to adulthood may contribute to the likelihood that an adolescent individual will continue to experiment with the drug (Mokrysz, Freeman, Korkki, & Curran, 2016).

Regardless of the underlying mechanisms that may mediate the prevalence of marijuana use during adolescence, the epidemiological evidence indicates a fair number of adolescent nervous systems are exposed to THC (Johnston et al., 2008). Thus, what impact does the THC have on the brain? With the presence of cannabinoid receptors in the cortex and hippocampal formation, chronic THC exposure, not surprisingly, can lead to myriad changes in cognition and emotionality (Pope et al., 2003; Rubino & Parolaro, 2008; Trezza, Cuomo, & Vanderschuren, 2008). Moreover, signaling through these receptors has been reported to have both neuroprotective and neurotoxic actions (Drysdale & Platt, 2003), so, again, it's not too shocking that THC (and THC-like chemicals) can have some profound effects on the structure and function of the brain (Chang, Yakupov, Cloak, & Ernst, 2006; Kolb, Gorny, Limebeer, & Parker, 2006; Lawston, Borella, Robinson, & Whitaker-Asmitia, 2000; Martin-Santos et al., 2010). However, as nothing in neurobiology is ever simple, the neurobiological effects of THC are also highly dependent on the age and sex of the individual, and the region of the brain considered, as well as the amount and exposure duration of THC and concurrent drug use (Jacobus et al., 2009; Weiland et al., 2015). Moreover, if this were not complicated enough, the body produces its own activators of the cannabinoid receptors, called the endocannabinoids, which have their own neuromodulatory roles (de Fonseca et al., 2004). Despite these complexities, we will attempt to summarize some of this burgeoning literature and try to shed some light on what THC might be doing to the adolescent brain and to a teenager's cognitive abilities.

From a gross, structural perspective, it appears the kids that started their marijuana use before they are 17 have smaller gray matter volumes, but larger white matter volumes, than kids that initiated use after they are 17 (Wilson et al., 2000). Remember, gray matter is the tissue in the brain where neurons make synaptic connections with one another, while white matter is made of the myelinated axonal tracts that connect bits of the brain together. Thus, a simple read of these data is that, overall, neuron-to-neuron communication may be compromised, but region-to-region transmission may be enhanced.

Another structural neuroimaging study showed changes in prefrontal cortical thickness in adolescent marijuana smokers, but these structural changes were region-specific, and not all in the same direction—there's that complexity again. Specifically, teenagers that smoke marijuana exhibit thinner insular and superior frontal cortices but thicker inferior parietal and superior temporal cortices, compared to nonsmoking teens (Lopez-Larson et al.,

2011). Although the exact functional ramifications of these previously mentioned hyperspecific structural changes are not completely understood, it is relatively safe to say that the adolescent brain can be physically shaped by THC exposure.

From a microscopic, cellular perspective, studies in adolescent animals have shown THC significantly alters the neurochemistry and function of neurons. For instance, one study found that intermittent THC exposure during the later stages of adolescence resulted in reduced levels of the naturally occurring opioids, and their receptors, in the nucleus accumbens and prefrontal cortex, compared to non-THC treated adolescent rats (Ellgren et al., 2008). It has also been shown that synthetic compounds that mimic THC also differentially affect the adult and adolescent brain. Specifically, a group of experimenters gave HU210, a synthetic cannabinoid, to both adult and adolescent rats for 14 days and then examined their brains 1 day later. These researchers found that adults chronically exposed to HU210 had fewer hippocampal $GABA_A$ receptors than their placebo-treated adult counterparts, while these same receptors were unaffected in adolescent animals whether or not they were treated with the THC-like drug (Verdurand, Dalton, & Zavitsanou, 2010). As $GABA_A$ receptors are integral in signaling inhibitory messages in neurons, these data suggest adult, but not adolescent, animals may exhibit reduced hippocampal excitability following chronic cannabinoid receptor stimulation.

Animal studies have also indicated that THC can alter hippocampal neurogenesis. In adult rats, for instance, chronic HU210 treatment results in an increase in neurogenesis in the dentate gyrus compared to adults not treated with HU210 (Jiang et al., 2005). Although little immediate effect of adolescent THC treatment has been reported on adolescent neurogenesis (Steel, Miller, Sim, & Day, 2014), adolescent male rats given HU210 show suppressed neurogenesis in adulthood, compared to adults not exposed to HU210 during adolescence (Lee, Wainwright et al., 2014). Interestingly, no effect of adolescent HU210 exposure on neurogenesis was found in adult females (Lee, Wainwright et al., 2014). Hence, adolescent exposure to THC and THC-like drugs influence neurogenesis, but these effects are dependent on when the exposure occurred, when neurogenesis is measured, and the sex of the animal (Figure 8.3).

The few previously mentioned studies indicate that marijuana can significantly affect the hippocampus. Thus, this begs the questions whether learning and memory are impaired in animals following exposure to THC

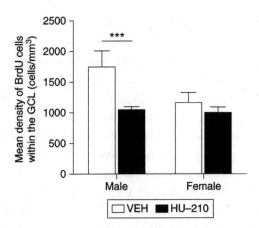

Figure 8.3. THC-like chemicals and neurogenesis in the dentate gyrus of adolescent-exposed males and females. The number of BrdU-positive cells in the sub-granular cell layer (GCL) of the dentate gyrus following exposure to the THC-like chemical HU-210 (black bars) or vehicle (white bars). Reprinted from T. T. Lee, S. R. Wainwright, M. N. Hill, L. A. M. Galea, & B. B. Gorzalka, 2014, Sex, drugs, and adult neurogenesis: Sex-dependent effects of escalating adolescent cannabinoid exposure on adult hippocampal neurogenesis, stress reactivity, and amphetamine sensitization, *Hippocampus 24*, 280–292. Used with permission from John Wiley and Sons, Inc.

and whether these impairments show any age dependence. The answer to both these questions appears to be yes, but it depends on variables such as the behavioral task and drug used. For example, although adolescent rats exposed to THC show poorer object recognition and spatial working memory compared to adults (Quinn et al., 2008; Steel, Miller, Sim, & Day, 2011), the synthetic cannabinoid, WIN 55212-2, does not appear to significantly affect spatial learning in either adolescent or adult animals (Acheson, Moore, Kuhn, Wilson, & Swartzwelder, 2011).

These types of studies assess the animals while they are adolescent *or* adult, but what happens to adults when they are exposed to marijuana *during* adolescence? That is, are there any long-term effects of cannabis on brain and behavior, and, if so, are any of these effects reversible? The bad news is that there do appear to be some lingering effects of adolescent THC exposure in adulthood, even after a long period of abstinence. Specifically, adolescent rats chronically treated with THC show impairments when tested in adulthood in a spatial memory test and a learning task that requires mental flexibility

(Harte & Dow-Edwards, 2010; Rubino et al., 2009). Moreover, these adult rats with prior THC experience also had fewer dendrites and dendritic spines on the neurons of their dentate gyrus compared to control rats (Rubino et al., 2009). Thus, in addition to the risk of adult psychotic disorders as alluded to in the beginning of this section (Andreasson et al., 1987; Arsenault et al., 2002; Malone et al., 2010), heavy cannabis use during adolescence may lead to long-term cognitive decrements as well. The good news, however, is that sustained abstinence from marijuana is associated with the reversal of some memory impairments, as well as functional reorganization of the brain (Chang et al., 2006; Schweinsburg et al., 2010). So it appears that while THC exposure during adolescent brain remodeling may not be ideal, it does appear THC/marijuana-induced changes in the brain are not necessarily hardwired and irreversible.

On a final note, it is important to point out that cannabis, in one form or another, has legitimate medicinal uses, particularly for neurological disorders (Gurley, Aranow, & Katz, 1998; Pryce & Baker, 2005; Robson, 2005; Wright, 2007). This leads to the quandary of whether an adolescent suffering from a condition that may be helped by cannabis would be better or worse off for taking it (Strang, Witton, & Hall, 2000). Like the complexities and intricacies that surround the effects of marijuana on adolescent brain in the first place, there is no one-size-fits-all solution to this problem. Suffice it to say, however, that depending on the health condition and the severity of such a condition, the adolescent individual, and their parent or guardian, would have to balance the possible pros and cons of medicinal cannabis use, like any other drug. It appears, however, from the previous reviewed literature, that at least the *recreational* use of marijuana would clearly be best kept to a minimum.

A "Nontraditional" Drug of Abuse: Adolescent Brain Remodeling on "Roids"

Anabolic-androgen steroids (AAS) are synthetic testosterone-like chemicals that have been effectively used in clinical settings for muscle wasting and severe weight loss associated with many chronic diseases (Basaria, Wahlstrom, & Dobs, 2001; Brower, 2002). However, people have figured out that using

AAS at much higher, supraphysiological doses can enhance their athletic performance and muscle-building potentials (Clark & Henderson, 2003). Although most people use AAS for these "cosmetic" purposes, animal research suggests that once use is initiated, AAS may become addictive (Sato, Schulz, Sisk, & Wood, 2008; Wood, 2004). Along these lines, it is interesting to note that, similar to other addictive drugs, emerging evidence indicates that testosterone affects the mesolimbic dopamine reward pathways in the brain (Packard, Cornell, & Alexander, 1997).

Unfortunately, the use of AAS by teenagers is on the rise (Bahrke, Yesalis, & Brower, 1998; Clark & Henderson, 2003). Given that hormones clearly contribute to the sculpting of the pubertal and adolescent brain (see Chapter 6) and that there are clear physical and psychological health consequences associated with AAS abuse in adults (reviewed in Hall, Hall, & Chapman, 2005; Kanayama, Hudson, & Pope, 2010; van Amsterdam, Opperhuizen, & Hartgens, 2010), we felt it would be appropriate to provide a brief review of what this troubling trend may mean to the maturation of the adolescent brain.

Epidemiological data point to an increase in the number of teenagers that abuse AAS, particularly among high school athletes. Specifically, estimates range from 4% to 12% in adolescent males and 0.5% to 2% in adolescent females (Bahrke et al., 1998; Rogol, 2010). Although there are many complexities that surround the use of AAS, such as type, dose, duration, and combination (i.e., "stacking") of the steroids taken, one common behavioral problem of teenagers that abuse AAS is an increase in aggression (Beaver, Vaughn, DeLisi, & Wright, 2008). Animal research, using a variety of species and tests of aggressive behavior, has also shown an association between pubertal AAS exposure and aggression (Farrell & McGinnis, 2004; Lumia & McGinnis, 2010; Ricci, Grimes, & Melloni, 2007; Salas-Ramirez, Montalto, & Sisk, 2008, 2010). These studies have also shown that even after adolescent AAS use is terminated, animals continue to show elevated levels of aggressive behavior in adulthood (Farrell & McGinnis, 2004; Grimes & Melloni, 2006; Grimes, Ricci, & Melloni, 2006; Salas-Ramirez et al., 2010).

There are a number of studies that have investigated the neurobiological mechanisms that underlie AAS-induced aggression during puberty (Melloni & Ricci, 2010). The brain areas that pop up regularly when perusing this literature are a group of interconnected nuclei in the hypothalamic and limbic regions, namely the anterior hypothalamus and lateral septum (Melloni & Ricci, 2010). For instance, following chronic AAS treatment, adolescent male hamsters show persistent neural activation in these nuclei (Ricci et al., 2007). These areas also show a whole host of neurochemical changes in response to adolescent AAS exposure, such as increases in dopaminergic (Ricci, Schwartzer, & Melloni, 2009), GABAergic (Grimes, Ricci, & Melloni, 2003), and vasopressinergic (DeLeon et al., 2002; Grimes et al., 2006) activity, with simultaneous decreases in glutamatergic (Carrillo, Ricci, & Melloni, 2009) and serotonergic (Grimes & Melloni, 2006) function. It is important to point out that as researchers have discovered these neurochemical alterations, they have been able to hone in on, and disrupt, some of these changes and reduce the aggressive behavior that happens with adolescent AAS use. For instance, animals treated with AAS along with drugs that enhance serotonergic activity show much less aggressive behavior than those animals only exposed to the AAS (Grimes & Melloni, 2002, 2005; Ricci, Rasakham, Grimes, & Melloni, 2006). These encouraging studies suggest that once neuroscientists figure out the complex changes wrought by adolescent AAS exposure, then they can attempt to reverse these effects by rebalancing an individual's neurochemistry.

In addition to these neurochemical experiments, there have also been some interesting studies investigating the effects of AAS on the structure of neurons and neurogenesis. Specifically, adolescent male rats treated with AAS during puberty showed an increase in dendritic spine density in both the amygdala and hippocampus compared to their nontreated counterparts (Cunningham, Claiborne, & McGinnis, 2007), suggesting greater excitatory signaling in these areas in the AAS-treated rats (Figure 8.4). In the context of neurogenesis, one study showed that AAS decreased hippocampal neurogenesis (Brannvall, Bogdanovic, Korhonen, & Lindholm, 2005), but as this study only looked at adult rats, it's unclear whether AAS affect neurogenesis during adolescence.

Although clearly more research needs to be done on how AAS use affects the adolescent brain, the literature to date points to many negative repercussions once the individual initiates use. So, in addition to trying to undo any unbalances caused by AAS in the teenage brain, it will be vitally important to keep teens from using AAS in the first place. Thus, similar to the other previously discussed abused drugs, an ounce of prevention may well be worth more than a pound of cure.

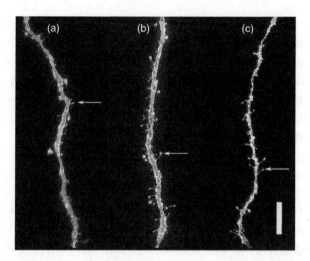

Figure 8.4. Anabolic steroids and morphology of amygdalar neurons in adolescent rats.
The morphology of dendrites and dendritic spines in the medial amygdala of male rats treated with (A) control, (B) androgenic anabolic steroids (AAS), or (C) AAS and given time to recover from the treatment (withdrawal). Scale bar = 10 μm. Reprinted from R. L. Cunningham, B. J. Claiborne, & M. Y. McGinnis, 2007, Pubertal exposure to anabolic androgenic steroids increases spine densities on neurons in the limbic system of male rats, *Neuroscience, 150,* 609–615. Used with permission from Elsevier.

Prescription Drugs and Adolescent Brain Remodeling

In the last part of this chapter, we turn to a couple of commonly used prescription drugs that may affect the developing brain more than we once thought. Specifically, we will discuss the selective serotonergic reuptake inhibitors (SSRIs; e.g., Prozac®, Zoloft®, Celera®, Paxil®) and methylphenidate (e.g., Ritalin®, Concerta®). These medications are largely prescribed to help combat depression and ADHD, respectively. Both these disorders show a relatively high prevalence rate during adolescence, with depression at about 15% to 20% and ADHD hovering around 9.5% to 13.5% (Centers for Disease Control, 2010; Cicchetti & Toth, 1998). Although the SSRIs and methylphenidate don't get as many newspaper headlines as the previously covered illicit drugs or drugs of abuse, these medications do have significant effects on the developing adolescent brain (Andersen & Navalta, 2004). However, before we discuss these effects, it is important to affirm that these prescription medications can, and under most conditions do, provide some relief to a number of individuals (and their families) dealing with adolescent depression and ADHD (Bridge, Salary, Birmaher, Asare, & Brent, 2005; Hechtman & Greenfield, 2003). Thus, unlike the previously reviewed abused drugs, these prescriptions drugs have a clear, Food and Drug Administration–approved medicinal purpose.

For the treatment of depression (and sometimes anxiety disorders), physicians often prescribe an SSRI such as Prozac*, Zoloft*, Celera*, or Paxil*. One simple neurochemical theory of depression is that there is not enough serotonin (5-HT) in the synapse (Stahl, 1992). Therefore, a rather straightforward treatment was designed to jack up the available 5-HT in the synapse by blocking its reuptake and metabolism (Vaswani, Linda, & Ramesh, 2003). As the acronym suggests, the SSRIs work by blocking the reuptake of 5-HT, although additional mechanisms are likely involved (Goodnick & Goldstein, 1998), and this simple strategy appears to be fairly successful in treating depression (Vaswani et al., 2003).

Following along this simple logical path, physicians also started to prescribe the SSRIs to depressed teenagers in an effort to relieve their symptoms of depression. However, an unfortunate side effect began to be noted in SSRI-treated adolescents, namely suicidal ideation (Hammad, Laughren, & Racoosin, 2006). Suicidal ideation is not suicide itself but, instead, suicidal thoughts, which can sometimes lead to a suicide attempt. It wasn't long until the Food and Drug Administration, as well as various European regulatory agencies, issued a statement that resulted in a "black box" warning on the package inserts to doctors and their patients that SSRIs increased the risk "of suicidal thinking and behavior (suicidality) in children, adolescents, and young adults." We bring this issue up not to condone or condemn the use of SSRIs in an adolescent psychiatric patient population, as there are many benefits and risks that are best weighed by the physician and patient (Bridge et al., 2005, 2007; Gibbons et al., 2007). We do, however, bring this up to make the important point (that hopefully is abundantly clear by this point in this book) that the adolescent brain is not just a smaller adult brain.

Regardless of the SSRI-adolescent-suicidality controversy, it is important to draw attention to the fact that 5-HT is also a major molder of the maturing nervous system (Frederick & Stanwood, 2009; Gaspar, Cases, & Maroteaux, 2003; Whitaker-Asmitia, 2001). Thus, surprise, surprise, SSRIs appear to have significant effects on the developing adolescent brain. For instance, PSA-NCAM levels, a proxy for synaptic plasticity, are elevated in the amygdala of adolescent rats in response to fluoxetine (Prozac°) treatment, while they are reduced in adults (Homberg et al., 2011), and paroxetine (Paxil°) exposure leads to greater activity in noradrenergic neurons in the adolescent than adult locus coeruleus (West, Ritchie, & Weiss, 2010). Another group of researchers showed that unlike the increase in neurogenesis in dentate gyrus of adult rats exposed to fluoxetine (Kodama, Fujioka, & Duman, 2004; Malberg, Eisch, Nestler, & Duman, 2000), adolescent animals do not show any fluoxetine-induced changes in neurogenesis (Hodes, Yang, van Kooy, Santollo, & Shors, 2009). Although this type of research is really just in its infancy, these few studies do clearly indicate that certain facets of the adolescent brain are differentially affected by SSRIs compared to the adult brain.

In addition to these age-dependent neurobiological effects, there are also behavioral differences in how adolescent and adult animals respond to SSRIs. One study showed that adolescent rats exhibited less wakefulness than adults following fluoxetine treatment (Homberg et al., 2011), while a separate experiment showed that rats given chronic fluoxetine during adolescence displayed changes in their performance on a visual discrimination task in adulthood (LaRoche & Morgan, 2007). Thus, along with the previously presented neurobiological data, it is clear that SSRIs have a distinctive impact on the behavior of an adolescent.

While the SSRIs act by upping the serotonergic tone of the depressed brain, methylphenidate acts by blocking the reuptake of dopamine to help reduce the scattered attention and hyperactivity characteristic of ADHD (Andersen, 2005; Kollins, 2008). Thus, methylphenidate works as a psychostimulant, similar to other dopamine reuptake inhibitors like cocaine (Volkow et al., 1995). Although it may seem counterintuitive to treat a hyperactive individual that has attention problems with a stimulant, it appears methylphenidate's efficacy is based on an inverted-U function. That is, if you treat individual A, who is operating at a low baseline activity level (left side of the inverted U), with a stimulant, thus increasing their stimulant concentration, this individual would experience an increase in activity (A'). This scenario appears to be responsible for the energy boost and cognitive enhancement non-ADHD individuals (i.e., person A') report when they take methylphenidate for these controversial purposes (Greely et al., 2008). However, if you treat individual B with a stimulant, and this individual is already operating at a high activity level (in the middle of the inverted U), then this ADHD-like individual experiences a decrease in activity following stimulant administration (B'; right side of the inverted U; Figure 8.5).

Independently of the paradoxical nature of using a stimulant to treat ADHD, methylphenidate does have significant effects on the structure and function of the developing adolescent brain, particularly in the meso-cortico-limbic reward system. For instance, following 2 weeks of methylphenidate exposure in adolescent male rats, there was increased expression of glial fibrillary acidic protein (GFAP), a marker of glial astrocytes, in the striatum and prefrontal cortex, as well as increases in the density of dendritic spines on the dendrites of prefrontal cortical neurons (Cavaliere et al., 2012). Similarly, male rats treated with methylphenidate through the neonatal to mid-pubertal periods of development show increased levels of markers of hippocampal structural plasticity (i.e., PSA-NCAM) and a greater number of cells in the prefrontal cortex, compared to controls (Gray et al., 2007). It is notable, however, that in this last study, most of these neurological changes return to the levels exhibited by controls once the animals reach adulthood (Gray et al., 2007). Although one study in rats showed that methylphenidate could briefly increase neurogenesis during adolescence (van der Marel et al., 2015), other studies have shown that methylphenidate given during

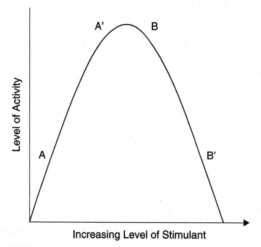

Figure 8.5. Inverted-U function and stimulant use.
An individual (A) operating at a low baseline activity level when treated with a stimulant will show an increase in their activity level (A'). However, an individual (B) operating at a high baseline activity levels treated with a stimulant will show a decrease in their activity levels (B').

adolescence leads to reduced hippocampal neurogenesis in adulthood, compared to those animals not exposed to the drug (Lagace, Yee, Bolanos, & Eisch, 2006; van der Marel et al., 2015). However, a different experiment conducted in adolescent male gerbils did not find a suppressive effect of methylphenidate on later adult neurogenesis (Schaefers, Teuchert-Noodt, Bagorda, & Brummelte, 2009), suggesting some species specificity to this effect of methylphenidate. Finally, methylphenidate administration for 1 week during adolescence in male rats has been reported to modulate the activity of dopamine neurons in the VTA such that a few days after methylphenidate withdrawal the activity of these neurons increases, while 2 weeks following withdrawal their activity levels decrease (Brandon, Marinelli, & White, 2003).

From a gene expression point of view, acute methylphenidate treatment in male rats in the throes of adolescence show increased expression of a variety of transcription factors and the genes important in opioid signaling in the striatum (Brandon et al., 2003). Interestingly, these effects of methylphenidate on striatal gene expression are potentiated by co-treatment with the SSRI fluoxetine (Waes, Beverley, Marinelli, & Steiner, 2010). These data suggest that when these medications are taken in combination, a not-uncommon occurrence in the growing number of adolescents with co-morbid depression and ADHD (Bhatara, Feil, Hoagwood, Vitiello, & Zima, 2004; Safer, Zito, & dosReis, 2003), they may have synergistic effects on neurobiological function.

In rats, chronic methylphenidate exposure during adolescence has been reported in some studies to impair and, in others, to improve performance on an assortment of learning and memory tasks (Heyser, Pelletier, & Ferris, 2004; LeBlanc-Duchin & Taukulis, 2007; Zhu, Weedon, & Dow-Edwards, 2007). So it remains unclear what exactly methylphenidate might be doing to an adolescent rat's ability to learn and remember information. There is also some behavioral evidence in rats that indicates that getting methylphenidate during puberty and then again in adulthood leads to changes in motor activity that are different than if they just get methylphenidate only in adulthood (Yang, Swann, & Dafny, 2010). Thus, there may be later changes in one's future sensitivity to methylphenidate once the original exposure has ended.

There are at least two clear conclusions that can be drawn from these few reviewed neurobiological and behavioral studies on methylphenidate. First, methylphenidate exposure during adolescence can significantly affect an individual's brain and behavior. Second, we need to do a whole lot more research if we want to truly understand the complex, and perhaps enduring, effects of methylphenidate on an adolescent's neurobehavioral function.

A very important caveat needs to be noted regarding these animal studies with both the SSRIs and methylphenidate. That is, the adolescent and adult animals treated with these drugs are not suffering from depression or ADHD. So, the results derived from these experiments may not necessarily represent what actually happens to a depressed or hyperactive teenage brain exposed to these medications for their intended purposes (Hyman, 2003). In fact, until biomedical researchers can develop animal models that faithfully recapitulate the neurobiological and physiological abnormalities seen in these disorders, it will be difficult to know the exact short- and long-term ramifications of these drugs on clinically depressed or hyperactive adolescent nervous systems. Another shortcoming of this area of basic research is that it is mainly conducted on male subjects. This may make some sense in the case of ADHD, which occurs more often in boys than girls (Cuffe et al., 2001), but makes less sense with depression, which shows a female-biased ratio (Kessler et al., 1994). Even with these limitations, however, the research conducted to date on psychotropic medication clearly indicates that adolescent and adult brains are differentially modulated in some specific and important ways.

Any Questions?

With these few examples of legal, illegal, and prescription drugs, we have tried to paint a picture, with very broad strokes, about the influence of drugs on the crucial remodeling project of the adolescent brain. As the number of teens that use, misuse, and abuse drugs show no signs of slowing, it will be imperative for doctors, parents, and, importantly, the teens themselves to understand the impact of drugs on the developing adolescent brain. Although the "any questions" part at the end of the PSA with the eggs and frying pan was surely rhetorical, there are still in fact many unanswered questions, and not just from a neuroscientific perspective, but from medical and societal perspectives as well.

For instance, what are the specific relationships between the structural and molecular changes in the brain induced by drugs and the changes in cognitive and emotional behavior observed in adolescents? Are these changes reversible and, if so, how? What are the best interventions to keep teens from abusing drugs in the first place, and what treatments might best mitigate any negative neurological or psychological consequences brought on by these drugs? At what age should certain drugs be legal, and should certain drugs never be made legal to begin with? We know it may sound like a conflict of interest from the authors of this book, both of whom are basic scientists, to simply state, "More research and funding are necessary," but, quite frankly, the costs, both in economic and personal terms, are much too high to let these questions go unanswered.

Recommended Reading

Degenhardt, L., Stockings, E., Patton, G., Hall, W. D., & Lynskey, M. (2016). The increasing global health priority of substance use in young people. *Lancet Psychiatry, 3,* 251–264.

Spear, L. P. (2016). Consequences of adolescent use of alcohol and other drugs: Studies using rodent models. *Neuroscience & Biobehavioral Reviews, 70,* 228–243.

Spear, L. P. (2018). Effects of adolescent alcohol consumption on the brain and behaviour. *Nature Reviews Neuroscience, 19,* 197–214.

9

Puberty and Adolescence in a Lifespan Context

If you have made it through the book to this point, we hope you have gained a better appreciation for the variety of psychobiological studies conducted on puberty and adolescence and the various levels of analysis used to interrogate this area of research. So far, we have tried to cover the basic neurobiological mechanisms that drive reproductive and behavioral maturation during this developmental period; the impact of various environmental factors, such as stress and drugs; the extent to which basic research informs our understanding of human adolescent development; and how research on human adolescents informs the direction of basic research. In this last chapter, we want to zoom out and look at puberty and adolescence from a broader societal perspective and ask what insights 21st-century research on puberty and adolescence might provide to those of us broadly interested in the ontogeny of human behavior.

The Adolescent Era

Adolescence is an era, alright. We usually remember our own adolescence as a distinct period fraught with the ups and downs of becoming an independent adult, and parents often think of their adolescent child as going through a phase that is sort of like the terrible twos, only a lot longer. In this section, we first attempt to define the opening and closing of the adolescent era and then ask whether this era of development spans a longer period than we thought, and, if so, does it matter for us as individuals and as a society.

The Adolescent Era Begins With the Onset
of Puberty and Ends With . . .

We will start with the easy one first. Almost by definition, the onset of puberty is the opening kickoff of adolescence because it marks the appearance of the very first indications that the body is transitioning to its adult morphology under the influence of gonadal hormones. Conveniently, we know when puberty occurs in an individual because we can *see* it. If you have read the previous chapters, then you know what happens next in terms of brain and behavioral development.

Now the hard one: How do we know when adolescence is done? How *would* we know when it is done? There are no overt signs of attainment of an adult brain analogous to those that signal the onset of adolescent brain development, and beyond that, it's not clear that even a neuroscientist would know an adult brain if they saw one. Sure, with longitudinal neuroimaging we might be able to determine a slight inflection point in the rate of cortical thinning that indicates some sort of transition from developmental thinning to plain old loss of gray matter that continues for the rest of your life (Peelle, Cusack, & Henson, 2012), but what makes us think that said inflection point marks the end of adolescence? Maybe it happens earlier than that, or maybe it happens later. Frankly, there is just no clear neural correlate of, or biomarker for, attainment of adulthood.

Part of the problem is that there is no good operational definition of *adult* or *adulthood* as applied to either brain or behavior, particularly if we agree that being an adult goes way beyond being capable of having children. Puberty is officially over once fertility is attained: Start to finish, this process does not take more than handful of years (Mendle, 2014), and as we mentioned earlier, virtually no one equates simply being fertile with being an adult. Along these lines, think about the decidedly fuzzy definition of adulthood in the United States as is used within our legal system or society. A person can join the armed forces at 17, can vote and consent to marry at 18, cannot buy cigarettes or alcohol until 21, but can stay on their parents' healthcare plan until they are 26. So for now, let us just say that the question of when the adolescent era ends is open for discussion, and that discussion will undoubtedly need to consider culture.

Is the Adolescent Era Experiencing Mission Creep?

The *teenage years* is commonly used shorthand for adolescence, but in reality, the adolescent era starts for most people a little before the teenage years and, by some biological and legal definitions, spills over into the 20s. However, has adolescence always been this long? Probably not. It seems that over the past 100 years or so, the adolescent period has been stretched out by being pulled at both ends; that is, the age at onset of puberty has become younger and the age at which individuals become independent of their families and take on full adult responsibilities has become older, at least in economically developed nations. Using the appearance of secondary sexual characteristics, such as breast and scrotal development as a marker for puberty, studies conducted in Europe and the United States find that the average age of puberty has advanced by ~1.5 years in both girls and boys, just in the last half of the 20th century (Herman-Giddens et al., 1997; Kaplowitz, Slora, Wasserman, Pedlow, & Herman-Giddens, 2001; Lee & Styne, 2013; Mendle, 2014; Figure 9.1). In the

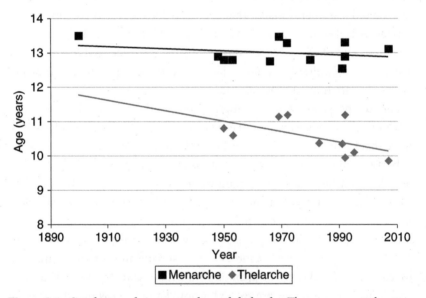

Figure 9.1. Secular trends in menarche and thelarche. There appears to be a trend with menarche (squares) and thelarche (diamonds) occurring earlier in girls. Reprinted from Y. Lee & D. Styne, 2013, Influences on the onset and tempo of puberty in human beings and implications for adolescent psychological development. *Hormones and Behavior, 64,* 250–261. Used with permission from Elsevier.

United States, the average age of menarche (first menstruation) decreased by ~2 years between the late 19th century and the mid-20th century (Wyshak & Frisch, 1982).

What is going on here? No doubt, part of the explanation is better nutrition and health in the 20th century compared to earlier times. However, there may be more nefarious influences too. Childhood obesity and exposure to endocrine disruptors, both 20th-century problems, may contribute to the secular trend in the earlier onset of puberty. For instance, we know fat cells can synthesize estradiol (Kershaw & Flier, 2004), and some endocrine disruptors mimic the effects of estrogens (Dickerson & Gore, 2007), and since breast development is an estrogen-dependent process, it may be that fat-derived estrogens and/or exposure to endocrine disruptors are resulting in a population-level decrease in the average age of breast development. Yet, remember from Chapter 2 that puberty is a brain event before it is a gonadal event, so early breast development resulting from obesity or exposure to endocrine disruptors would not reflect "true" puberty. In contrast, menarche does require hormonal release driven by the brain, indicating "true" puberty is occurring earlier. However, the decrease in age at menarche observed between the 19th and 20th centuries leveled off in the mid-20th century. So one possibility is that improved nutrition and health may account for the decrease in age at menarche, and we have hit the lower limit of how young fertility can be achieved as selected for during human evolution. Gluckman and colleagues make this precise argument (Gluckman & Hanson, 2006b). During the millennia and centuries when nutrition and health were not so good, they posit that the age at onset of puberty was actually pushed back, and all we are witnessing now is a return to the (younger) age of pubertal onset that is evolutionarily normal for humans.

What about secular trends in the age at completion of adolescence? Since we have not had (and still do not have) any good biological markers for the end of adolescence, it is impossible to document whether adolescence is finished at later ages now as compared with centuries ago. To be sure, 21st-century imaging studies tell us that human adolescent brain development is a more protracted process than 20th-century neuroscientists ever imagined. However, was Sol Bloom, who at the age of 20 masterminded the Midway Plaisance at the 1893 Chicago World's Columbian Exposition, still suffering from an immature prefrontal cortex? Moreover, going back to the point that, in the United States, we cannot make up our minds when an individual is legally an adult anyway, we wonder whether culture, and not basic human biology, explains why the prefrontal cortex does not get its act completely together until age 25. Our own suspicion is that contemporary culture has lowered expectations for when an adolescent is supposed to step up to the plate and start functioning as an adult in society. Perhaps as a society, we are giving 18-year-olds the permission and luxury of spending 7 more years as dependents. Experience is a powerful shaper of synaptic plasticity, so it makes sense that if full adult responsibilities were thrust upon one at 18 or 20 years of age, as was the case not that long ago, then prefrontal cortex would have to sit up straight and pay attention relatively sooner. Longitudinal imaging of the brain of 10- to 25-year-olds growing up in the 1800s could shed some light on this speculation, but since that is impossible, we perhaps could settle for cross-cultural studies that compare the trajectory of adolescent brain development in populations in which adult responsibilities (e.g., financial independence, parenthood) are assumed at younger versus older ages. It might also be interesting to compare adolescent brain development within a culture, for example, individuals who join the military or become parents at 17 years of age versus those who do not assume these adult responsibilities until 25 years of age. Answers to these questions, however, remain unknown.

Implications of a Lengthening Adolescent Era

No matter the reasons, it is a reality that in economically developed societies, the number of years between the onset of puberty and attainment of adulthood is longer than it has ever been. We have just discussed this as a function of trends in puberty occurring earlier and functioning independently as an adult occurring later. Another way to look at this situation is that it creates a mismatch between biological (reproductive) maturation and psychosocial maturation. Gluckman and Hanson (2006) argue that this mismatch is occurring for the first time in human evolution (Figure 9.2). That is, in the hunter-gatherer period 20,000 years ago, puberty and psychosocial maturation occurred relatively early, but simultaneously, so that individuals were assuming adult responsibilities in these societies by 15 or 16 years of age. Then, fast-forwarding to the Roman Empire some 2,000 years ago or the later stages of the Industrial Revolution 200 years ago, undernutrition, childhood disease, and poor hygiene resulted in a later onset of puberty, but society had become more complex and so the age of psychosocial maturation was also pushed back. It is only recently, with better nutrition and modern medical

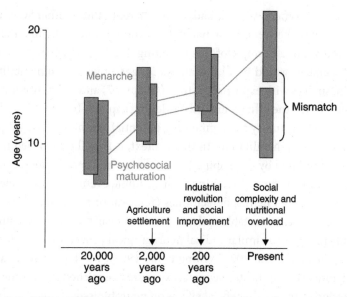

Figure 9.2. Mismatch between menarche and psychological maturity. The theoretical association and apparent mismatch between the onset of menarche (dark grey bars) and attainment of psychological maturity (light grey bars) in girls throughout history. Reprinted from P. D. Gluckman & M. A. Hanson, 2006, Evolution, development and timing of puberty, *Trends in Endocrinology and Metabolism, 17,* 7–12. Used with permission from Elsevier.

control of childhood disease, that the onset of puberty is reverting to the younger age that it was originally selected for, but the world is more complex than ever, and it is not expected that someone should be able to function as an independent adult until their mid-20s.

In fact, these loosening societal expectations have even led to the proposition of yet another phase of human development dubbed "emerging adulthood" (Arnett, 2000), roughly associated with the 18- to 25-year-old age range—that grey zone of not really being an adolescent anymore, but not having assumed the responsibilities of independent adulthood either. Whether or not emerging adulthood is a unique, distinct stage of human development sandwiched between adolescence and adulthood is a matter of debate among developmental psychologists (Cote, 2014). In any case, this construct applies primarily to individuals in developed, economically advanced countries and brings us back to the notion that the end of adolescence is a sociocultural, not biological, construct.

Is this phenomenon good, bad, or indifferent? Put another way: Is this elongated glass half-empty or half-full? Although questions like these are often relative, one example of this widening developmental stage as a half-empty scenario would be that it allows longer times for vulnerabilities to creep in, such as with exposure to stress (Chapter 7) and brain-altering drugs (Chapter 8). On the other hand, this widening gap may be viewed as a longer window of opportunity for augmenting potential for the positive influences of intervention/rehabilitation. In this context, it is well established that the plasticity exhibited by developing brains allows for a certain degree of resilience, even in the face of seemingly catastrophic events. For example, children who undergo hemispherectomies (removal of one hemisphere of the brain) for severe, intractable epilepsy can lead near normal lives compared to adults receiving a similar radical neurosurgical procedure (Pulsifer et al., 2004; Spencer & Huh, 2008; Vining et al., 1997). Moreover, there is a sizable literature that indicates neonatal exposure to enriched environments for long periods can have beneficial effects on neurobiological function, such as increased cortical thickness, neural connectivity, and neurogenesis (Mora, Segovia, & del Arco, 2007). So, does the protracted maturation of the adolescent brain lend similar protective plasticity and the ability to benefit from enriching environments? Fortunately, this half-full scenario appears to be the case.

One striking example comes from a study where the experimenters made lesions of the medial preoptic area (mPOA) in prepubertal rats (Twiggs, Popolow, & Gerall, 1978). This brain region is crucially important in the display of male sexual behavior, such that adults bearing mPOA lesions show irreversible deficits in mating behavior (Christensen, Nance, & Gorski, 1977). Not surprisingly, rats in this study given mPOA lesions prior to puberty were unable to show reproductive behaviors upon reaching adulthood (Twiggs et al., 1978). The interesting twist was that some of the animals with mPOA lesions were raised in social groups during adolescence, and remarkably, these socially living animals were able to demonstrate mating behaviors as adults (Twiggs et al., 1978). Therefore, this elegant study indicates that adolescence and a specific type of social environment can interact to ameliorate or even reverse prior brain damage.

Also, recall from Chapter 7 that animals exposed to enriched environments during adolescence following significant episodes of prenatal or neonatal stress show physiological and behavioral phenotypes strikingly similar to animals that have not experienced prenatal or neonatal adversity (Bredy,

Humpartzoomian, Cain, & Meaney, 2003; Bredy, Zhang, Grant, Diorio, & Meaney, 2004; Francis, Diorio, Plotsky, & Meaney, 2002; Morley-Fletcher, Rea, Maccari, & Laviola, 2003). These lines of research would suggest that the developmental mechanisms making the adolescent brain sensitive to environmental inputs might make vulnerability and resilience two sides of the same coin. Therefore, in the end, this expanding glass may be growing half-emptier *and* half-fuller.

The Timing of Puberty, Psychosocial Development, and Psychopathology

Puberty and adolescence are associated with increased prevalence of mental illnesses, some of which affect one sex more than the other, including mood and anxiety disorders, eating disorders, substance use disorders, and psychoses (Lee, Heimer et al., 2014). These illnesses may be relatively rare in children simply because we typically go to great lengths to protect them from the inconvenient truths of adulthood until they are mentally and socially able to understand them. However, the well-established association between the onset of puberty and increased risk of psychopathology raises the question of whether early or late bloomers are at greater or lesser risk for psychopathologies associated with adolescence, and, if so, does sex matter?

The relationship between pubertal timing and risk of psychopathology is exceedingly difficult to sort out for a number of reasons. First, complex (and not well-understood) interactions between genes, hormones, brain development, and experience ultimately determine how healthy an individual is when they emerge from the adolescent era. Second, genetic and environmental variables are often confounded, and both can influence the timing of puberty. Third, merely showing the physical signs of puberty profoundly changes one's experiences, and if these signs appear much earlier or much later than peers, then this mistiming is likely to affect interactions with both peers and adults. In fact, off-time maturation could be considered as an additional stressor or vulnerability that interacts with pre-existing biological risk factors, and even this may be exacerbated if elevated hormones increase sensitivity to environmental conditions.

It will come as no surprise that the answer to the question of whether off-time puberty alters risk for psychopathology is complicated, not entirely clear, and does depend on sex. The reader is referred to recent reviews for a more comprehensive look at the literature (Dimler & Natsuaki, 2015; Galvao et al., 2014; Golub et al., 2008; Graber, 2013; Klump, 2013; Mendle, Turkheimer, & Emery, 2007; Trotman et al., 2013), but we'll try to simplify and briefly summarize the best documented effects noted in these reviews. Let us start with girls. Early puberty in girls is associated with higher rates of both internalizing and externalizing symptoms and with higher rates of disorders, including depression, substance use, disruptive behavior, and eating disorders, with some studies showing persistence into adulthood. Studies of pubertal timing and eating disorders in girls are particularly consistent in finding an association between both early pubertal timing and advanced stage of puberty with higher rates of disordered eating symptoms, and these effects seem to persist into young adulthood. Interestingly, late puberty in girls does not appear to be a problem and may actually confer some advantages, as academic achievement is better in late maturing girls. For boys, early puberty is associated with elevated internalizing and externalizing symptoms in early and mid-adolescence, but there is not much evidence for either persistence of elevated symptoms or effects on prevalence of disorders. In contrast, late maturation in boys is linked to elevated risk for conduct and substance use disorders in young adulthood (although conclusions are qualified by relatively small effect sizes found in the studies). Finally, it is of interest to note that mistimed puberty is not associated with prevalence of psychotic disorders in either girls or boys, but gonadal hormones seem to modulate symptomatology, with low levels of both estrogen and testosterone associated with less symptoms.

Gender Dysphoria

Many individuals whose gender identity does not match the sex they were assigned at birth (i.e., transgender) experience distress, anxiety, and depression to such an extent that they meet diagnostic criteria for gender dysphoria (American Psychological Association, 2013). Gender dysphoria in children is particularly problematic for parents and healthcare providers in deciding whether some sort of treatment is necessary, because gender identity can be fluid in young individuals, and, on average, they usually outgrow it. Current estimates are that fewer than 25% of people with a childhood diagnosis of gender dysphoria continue as gender dysphoric in adolescence (Berenbaum & Beltz, 2011; Byne et al., 2012; Steensma, Kreukels, de Vries,

& Cohen-Kettenis, 2013). Yet, what is a parent to do if gender dysphoria is persistent as the child approaches puberty? In these cases, the recommendation by the medical profession has often been to suspend the onset of puberty by treatment with a long-acting GnRH receptor agonist, which desensitizes the pituitary to GnRH, prohibiting gonadotropin secretion and gonadal maturation (see Chapter 2). Delaying puberty in gender dysphoric children is thought to be beneficial for several reasons. First, the trauma of experiencing the physical changes (e.g., secondary sex characteristic) of a "wrong" puberty is like applying salt to the wound of someone already dealing with the psychological distress caused by the incongruence of their body and their gender identity. Second, because there is some evidence that gender identity is consolidated during adolescence, delay of puberty allows for some additional time for sorting things out. Finally, if an individual eventually does elect to live their life as their preferred gender and opt for cross-sex hormone treatment or gender reassignment surgery, then the transsexual process is more easily accomplished if the body and brain are still in a prepubertal state, unencumbered by the activational and organizational influences of gonadal hormones (see Chapter 6).

However, what if gender dysphoria eventually desists in an individual in which puberty has been put on hold, and they end up with a body and gender identity that are congruent? Have they missed out on important influences of gonadal hormones if puberty doesn't occur until later or after the sensitive period for hormonal organization of the adolescent brain? Maybe, but it's important to remember that most of what we know about organizational effects of gonadal hormones during puberty is based on research in laboratory animals that are not exposed during adolescent development to the social and cultural experiences typical of human teenagers, independent of whether their teenage brains are being bathed in hormones. Thus, social experiences in humans could mitigate any adverse consequences of the absence of gonadal hormones during adolescence, whether that absence is due to naturally occurring or medically induced delayed puberty. The animal literature suggests that the absence of gonadal hormones during adolescent brain development mostly affects social behaviors and social cognition. If that generalizes to humans, then postponement of puberty in gender dysphoric children could have some consequences on social interactions in adulthood, but these potential consequences would have to be weighed with how gender dysphoria itself could influence social interactions. These tough unanswered questions may have been part of the reason a recent set of clinical practice guidelines put forth by the Endocrine Society suggested not to block the onset of puberty in children with gender dysphoria (Hembree et al., 2017), with a more wait-and-see approach, and then honor the requests for suppression of puberty if an adolescent requests such treatment.

Another thing to consider in this context is whether the GnRH agonists used to postpone puberty have direct effects on adolescent brain development, independent of the suppression of gonadal hormone secretion, given that GnRH receptors are expressed in various brain regions, including in the hypothalamus, amygdala, and prefrontal cortex (Jennes, Dalati, & Conn, 1988). Recent research in sheep provides some evidence for this possibility. Male sheep treated with a GnRH agonist during puberty and tested for spatial learning and memory after discontinuation of the agonist showed impairments in long-term spatial memory that persisted for several months to a year (Hough, Bellingham, Haraldsen, McLaughlin, Robinson et al., 2017). These impairments were also seen in sheep that received testosterone replacement during the time of GnRH agonist treatment, suggesting a direct and long-lasting effect of GnRH agonist on long-term spatial memory independent of suppression of testosterone (Hough, Bellingham, Haraldsen, McLaughlin, Rennie et al., 2017). Clearly, there is a lot left to be sorted out regarding the thorny question of postponement of puberty in gender dysphoric children, but at this point, research unfortunately gives parents and physicians very little to go on in weighing the costs and benefits.

Is Adolescent Brain Development Experience-Expectant or Experience-Dependent?

To answer whether adolescent brain development is experience-expectant or experience-dependent, let's start by generally defining these things (Greenough, Black, & Wallace, 1987). If we think about the relationship between experience and the nervous system in very broad terms, it boils down to the notion that experience results in the encoding of environmental information within neural circuits. Then we can think about two categories of environmental information or experience. The first category is environmental information that is ubiquitous for all individuals of a given species throughout most of its evolution; in the absence of this information, normal development does not occur. Two examples of experience-expectant development in humans are the requirement for visual sensory experience for normal wiring of visual cortex and binocular vision (Hensch, 2005) and exposure to spoken words for normal acquisition of oral language (Robinson, 1998). In other words, experience-expectant development of neural circuits involves a critical period during which the experience *must* occur; otherwise, the underlying function is severely impaired.

The second category is environmental information that is unique to a particular individual and sculpts neural circuits in a more refined way. Examples of experience-dependent development include exposure to one's native language, and growing up in an enriched or impoverished environment. Experience-dependent development does not involve a well-defined critical period, although there may well be certain times during development that a particular experience exerts more profound influences than at others; such times are more accurately described as *sensitive* periods, and not critical periods.

Can we neatly categorize adolescent brain development as either experience-expectant or experience-dependent? At first glance, it might seem obvious that adolescence is experience-dependent, because it is hard to come up with an experience that *must* occur during that time to create a functional adult brain, and conversely, it is easy to come up with experiences that shape the trajectory of adolescent brain development. However, there is one adolescent experience that has been ubiquitous for all humans throughout our evolution, and that is the appearance of gonadal hormones during puberty. Therefore, by that relatively strict definition then adolescence could be thought of as an experience-expectant developmental period during which the absence of gonadal hormonal influences would result in seriously compromised maturation of neural circuits underlying social behaviors. If you have a hard time buying the notion that the pubertal elevation in gonadal hormones is an experience, then you might have an easier time considering social play as an example of a sensory experience that is expected by the adolescent nervous system and required for normal maturation of social cognition and social skills (Bell, Pellis, & Kolb, 2010).

Nevertheless, the data that are out there suggest that adolescence is *not* an experience-expectant critical period of development during which the absence of exposure to gonadal hormones would totally incapacitate an individual. Instead, it appears that adolescence is an experience-dependent sensitive period for influences of gonadal hormones on brain and behavioral development. Recall from Chapter 6 that when male rodents are gonadectomized prior to the onset of puberty, and therefore deprived of gonadal hormones during adolescence, they are perfectly capable of expressing social behaviors such as sex and aggression in adulthood. However, they are socially awkward and seem to have trouble interpreting social cues received from conspecifics, so it appears that gonadal hormones program aspects of social cognition and behavioral flexibility and not social behavior per se. Experiments of nature in humans point to the same idea. For example, men with congenital hypogonadotropic hypogonadism do not undergo a natural puberty and typically do not begin testosterone replacement therapy until 17 years of age or older, effectively resulting in much of their adolescent development occurring in the absence of testicular hormones. Once on testosterone replacement therapy, these men can have sexual relationships, but report long-lasting psychosexual problems, such as difficulty with intimate relationships and body image concerns (Dwyer, Quinton, Pitteloud, & Morin, 2015). Research in animals and humans, therefore, tells us that the trajectory of adolescent maturation of social cognition certainly depends on, and is influenced by, gonadal hormones, but the adolescent social brain does not expect, and does not require, gonadal hormones for adult social behaviors to be expressed.

Research in animals and humans also supports the notion that adolescence is a sensitive period for these influences of gonadal hormones on social behavior; that is, hormones have a greater effect on the nervous system and behavior during adolescence than they do in adulthood. In fact, it appears that the end of adolescence (whenever that is) marks the closing of a postnatal period of sensitivity to organizational influences of gonadal hormones. For example, if animals are gonadectomized during early postnatal life and then receive a 3-week period of testosterone replacement therapy before, during, or after the normal time of puberty and adolescence, testosterone replacement normalizes male sexual behavior only if given before or during adolescence, and not if given after (Schulz, Molenda-Figueira, & Sisk, 2009).

In humans, adolescence seems to be a sensitive period for hormonal influences on spatial ability, for which men, on average, are better than women (Hampson, 1995). Both late maturing men and men with hypogonadotropic hypogonadism during the normal time of puberty perform more poorly on tests of spatial cognition than early maturing men or men who acquired hypogonadotropic hypogonadism in adulthood (Beltz & Berenbaum, 2013; Hier & Crowley, 1982). These studies provide evidence for relative insensitivity of the adult brain to effects of testosterone on both social and nonsocial behaviors that are organized by testosterone during puberty. It is not so clear about adolescence as a sensitive period for effects of ovarian hormones in women, although no effects of pubertal timing on verbal or spatial ability were detected in women in the same study that showed such an effect on spatial ability in men (Beltz & Berenbaum, 2013).

One way to think about all of this business regarding the role of experience during adolescent development is the concept of metaplasticity: the plasticity of plasticity. It might be hard to wrap your brain around this concept at first, but it helps to consider other "metas." Meta-analysis is an analysis of analyses. Meta-cognition, as famously explained by Donald Rumsfeld, is "There are known knowns; . . . things we know that we know. We also know there are known unknowns; . . . things that we know we don't know." Thus, metaplasticity is the plasticity of plasticity. At the cellular level, metaplasticity entails a change in the physiological or biochemical state of neurons or synapses that alters their ability to generate synaptic plasticity later (Abraham, 2008). As applied to adolescent development, metaplasticity means that the history of activity of neural circuits during adolescence, such as the experiences that are encountered, can make these same circuits either more or less plastic in adulthood. Metaplasticity during adolescence results in some paradoxical outcomes that, at first blush, can be hard to digest. Take, for example, the organizational effects of pubertal testosterone on male social behaviors and social cognition that were discussed at length in Chapter 6. When a neural circuit is organized by testosterone, by definition the circuit becomes less plastic than it was before the organizing action. Yet one of the long-lasting organizational effects of testosterone on behavior is to render the male rodent more flexible during social encounters and better able to adapt his behavior as a result of social experience. How could testosterone gel a circuit during adolescence in a way that makes that circuit seemingly more plastic in social situations later in adulthood? We are still working on that.

Where Do We Go From Here?

As we have noted throughout the chapters of this book, many questions remain unanswered. However, here at the end of this last chapter, we would like to draw attention to a few caveats and issues relevant to how one studies adolescent neurobehavioral maturation. We hope that keeping these matters in mind will help push the field forward or at least nudge the blinds open a bit more, to shine a little more light on the subject.

The first chapter of this book remarked on the significant uptick in neurobehavioral research over the last couple of decades devoted to better understanding adolescent development. Of course, it is all about us humans, but we rely on animal models for experimental control to infer causal relationships, discovery of neurobiological mechanisms, and study of biological variables isolated from psychosocial and cultural variables. But therein lies the problem: Humans grow up in societies and cultures that provide powerful experiences. Sometimes these experiences ameliorate adverse influences of a biological variable, and sometimes they exacerbate them. We can never recapitulate the human condition in laboratory animals, and that limits their use and generalizability in our quest to understand puberty and adolescence. However, animal models are our best bet for controlled experiments, and we should be OK as along as we are mindful of the inherent limitations and design experiments that take into consideration the natural history and ecology of the species that is studied.

One obvious difference is the length of time it takes a human (years) versus some rodents (weeks) to transition through adolescence, with clear drawbacks in the context of limiting the experiences and length of manipulations used in nonhuman animal experiments—but with the advantage of being able to answer mechanistic questions in a much shorter period. Yet, with these caveats in mind, some of the similarities between nonhuman animals and humans might surprise us. For example, as mentioned in Chapter 5, teenagers are notoriously influenced by the presence of peers, and they will take much more risk when peers are present than when alone (Gardner & Steinberg, 2005). It would appear that this example of social influence is unique to humans, but maybe not. It turns out that adolescent mice consume more alcohol in the presence of peers, but adult mice do not (Logue, Chein, Gould, Holliday, & Steinberg, 2014), so perhaps there is more to the "simple experimental animal model" than meets the eye. Nevertheless, the relative lack of psychosocial and cultural variables in many nonhuman animal studies, and the length of these developmental processes in general, need to be appreciated when researchers discuss the implications of their data in the context of human adolescence.

Regardless of the human or nonhuman nature of the experimental subject, great progress continues to be made in deepening our understanding of adolescent neurobehavioral development. Moving forward, however, it might benefit the research if experimenters, when possible, added variables or different levels of analysis to their experimental designs. For instance, many research designs meant to investigate neurobiological function in the adolescent brain will compare one group of adolescents to another group of adolescents, say adolescent mice exposed to alcohol or not. If alcohol has an effect on the adolescent brain, then the conclusion is often drawn that alcohol affects area "X" of the adolescent brain. However, if this previously mentioned experimental design were to use additional groups of adult mice exposed to the same conditions as the adolescence mice, then the research would be able to establish whether the effects of alcohol on brain area "X" were *specific* to adolescence. That is, does alcohol affect this area of the brain only during adolescence, or is this effect of alcohol something that happens to this brain area independent of when the exposure occurs? Of course, it is not always feasible to add to one's experimental design, due to laboratory space, time, and/or budget constraints, but when possible it could enrich a data set to answer not just whether the adolescent brain is or is not sensitive to a variable, but whether it is *especially* sensitive to that variable.

Along these lines, when studying adolescent subjects, it would be ideal if different segments of adolescent development are included in the experimental design. For example, if one studies impulse control in a go–no-go task, it would be best to determine not only if impulse control changes in adolescent subjects, but also the trajectory of this change across adolescent development. As we have seen throughout the experiments described in these chapters, the journey may just be as interesting as the destination. Again, there might be many valid reasons why adding experimental groups to afford this type of temporal resolution may not be possible in any given study, but the payoff in the end might be well worth the time and effort.

Finally, as we have alluded to in many of the chapters, it will be imperative to include both sexes in experimental designs, not only because of profound differences in past and present hormonal exposures, but equally profound experiential differences in periadolescent males and females. This will surely be aided by the new National Institutes of Health initiative of mandating the consideration of sex as a biological variable in experimental designs. This mandate should at least get many experimenters to become more cognizant of these hormonal differences between the sexes, as well as the hormonal differences within an individual over time, including the effects of estrous or menstrual cycles, circadian influences, or position in the pecking order, factors known to influence hormone levels profoundly (Nelson, 2011).

Obviously, these are only a few general suggestions, and as new techniques and methods become available to study adolescent maturation, experimental designs and analyses will need to evolve in parallel. However, taking these few issues into consideration when designing an experiment could provide even greater amounts of information as well as make one's conclusions more generalizable and impactful, which we can all agree in this context: More is better.

The Immense Unknown

As we conclude this book, we would like to quote from the French polymath Pierre-Simon Laplace, who supposedly muttered on his deathbed in 1827, "What we know is not much. What we do not know is immense." We feel this accurately sums up the current state of our understanding of the neurobiology and psychobiology of puberty and adolescence. To be sure, this tip-of-the-iceberg problem should not discourage us from diving deeper into the unknown. Instead, we hope these unknowns will drive and push us to continue to chip away at this immense unknown.

Literature Cited

Abraham, W. C. (2008). Metaplasticity: Tuning synapses and networks for plasticity. *Nature Reviews Neuroscience, 9,* 387–399.

Abreu-Villaca, Y., Seidler, F. J., Tate, C. A., & Slotkin, T. A. (2003). Nicotine is a neurotoxin in the adolescent brain: Critical periods, patterns of exposure, regional selectivity, and dose thresholds for macromolecular alterations. *Brain Research, 979,* 114–128.

Acheson, S. K., Moore, N. L. T., Kuhn, C. M., Wilson, W. A., & Swartzwelder, H. S. (2011). The synthetic cannabinoid WIN 55212-2 differentially modulates thigmotaxis but not spatial learning in adolescent and adult animals. *Neuroscience Letters, 487,* 411–414.

Adolphs, R. (2001). The neurobiology of social cognition. *Current Opinions in Neurobiology, 11,* 231–239.

Adriani, W., & Laviola, G. (2003). Elevated levels of impulsivity and reduced place conditioning with d-amphetamine: Two behavioral features of adolescence in mice. *Behavioral Neuroscience, 117,* 695–703.

Ahima, R. S., Dushay, J., Flier, S. N., Prabakaran, D., & Flier, J. S. (1997). Leptin accelerates the onset of puberty in normal female mice. *Journal of Clinical Investigation, 99,* 391–395.

Ahmed, E. I., Zehr, J. L., Schulz, K. M., Lorenz, B. H., DonCarlos, L. L., & Sisk, C. L. (2008). Pubertal hormones modulate the addition of new cells to sexually dimorphic brain regions. *Nature Neuroscience, 11,* 995–997.

Alaux-Cantin, S., Warnault, V., Legastelois, R., Botia, B., Pierrefiche, O., Vilpoux, C., & Naassila, M. (2013). Alcohol intoxications during adolescence increase motivation for alcohol in adult rats and induce neuroadaptations in the nucleus accumbens. *Neuropharmacology, 67,* 521–531.

Albert, D. J., & Walsh, M. L. (1984). Neural systems and the inhibitory modulation of agonistic behavior: A comparison of mammalian species. *Neuroscience and Biobehavioral Reviews, 8,* 5–24.

Alexander-Bloch, A., Giedd, J. N., & Bullmore, E. (2013). Imaging structural co-variance between human brain regions. *Nature Reviews Neuroscience, 14,* 322–336.

Altman, J. (1969). Autoradiographic and histological studies of postnatal neurogenesis. IV. Cell proliferation and migration in the anterior forebrain, with special reference to persisting neurogenesis in the olfactory bulb. *Journal of Comparative Neurology, 137,* 433–457.

American Psychological Association. (2004). Amicus curiae brief filed in U.S. Supreme Court in Roper v. Simmons. 543 U.S. 551 (2005).

American Psychiatric Association (2013). *Diagnostic and statistical manual of mental disorders* (5th ed.). Arlington, VA: .

Andersen, S. L. (2003). Trajectories of brain development: Point of vulnerability or window of opportunity. *Neuroscience and Biobehavioral Reviews, 27,* 3–18.

Andersen, S. L. (2005). Stimulants and the developing brain. *Trends in Pharmacological Sciences, 26,* 237–243.

Andersen, S. L., & Navalta, C. P. (2004). Altering the course of neurodevelopment: A framework for understanding the enduring effects of psychotropic drugs. *International Journal of Developmental Neuroscience, 22,* 423–440.

Andersen, S. L., Thompson, R. F., Krenzel, E., & Teicher, M. H. (2002). Pubertal changes in gonadal hormones do not underlie adolescent dopamine receptor overproduction. *Psychoneuroendocrinology, 27,* 683–691.

Andreasson, S., Allebeck, P., Engstrom, A., & Rydberg, U. (1987). Cannabis and schizophrenia: A longitudinal study of Swedish conscripts. *Lancet, 330,* 1483–1486.

Andrews, T. J., Halpern, S. D., & Purves, D. (1997). Correlated size variations in human visual cortex, lateral geniculate, and optic tract. *Journal of Neuroscience, 17,* 2859–2868.

Arnett, J. J. (1999). Adolescent storm and stress, reconsidered. *American Psychologist, 54,* 317–326.

Arnett, J. J. (2000). Emerging adulthood: A theory of development from the late teens through the twenties. *American Psychologist, 55,* 469–480.

Arnett, J. J. (2006). G. Stanley Hall's adolescence: Brilliance and nonsense. *History of Psychology, 9,* 186–197.

Arsenault, L., Cannon, M., Poulton, R., Murray, R., Caspi, A., & Moffitt, T. E. (2002). Cannabis use in adolescence and risk for adult psychosis: Longitudinal prospective study. *British Medical Journal, 325,* 1212–1213.

Bahrke, M. S., Yesalis, C. E., & Brower, K. J. (1998). Anabolic-androgenic steroid abuse and performance-enhancing drugs among adolescents. *Child and Adolescent Psychiatric Clinics of North America, 7,* 821–838.

Baker, B. L., Dermody, W. C., & Reel, J. R. (1975). Distribution of gonadotropin-releasing hormone in the rat brain as observed with immunocytochemistry. *Endocrinology, 97,* 125–135.

Barash, I. A., Cheung, C. C., Weigle, D. S., Ren, H., Kabigting, E. B., Kuijper, J. L., ... Steiner, R. A. (1996). Leptin is a metabolic signal to the reproductive system. *Endocrinology, 137,* 3144–3147.

Barha, C. K., Brummelte, S., Lieblich, S. E., & Galea, L. A. M. (2011). Chronic restraint stress in adolescence differentially influences hypothalamic–pituitary–adrenal axis function and adult hippocampal neurogenesis in male and female rats. *Hippocampus, 21,* 1216–1227.

Basaria, S., Wahlstrom, J. T., & Dobs, A. S. (2001). Clinical Review 138: Anabolic-androgenic steroid therapy in the treatment of chronic diseases. *Journal of Clinical Endocrinology and Metabolism, 86,* 5108–5117.

Baum, M. J. (1979). Differentiation of coital behavior in mammals: A comparative analysis. *Neuroscience and Biobehavioral Reviews, 3,* 265–284.

Bava, S., & Tapert, S. F. (2010). Adolescent brain development and the risk for alcohol and other drug problems. *Neuropsychology Review, 20,* 398–413.

Beaver, K. M., Vaughn, M. G., DeLisi, M., &Wright, J. P. (2008). Anabolic-androgenic steroid use and involvement in violent behavior in a nationally representative sample of young adult males in the United States. *American Journal of Public Health, 98,* 2185–2187.

Becker, J. B., & Hu, M. (2008). Sex differences in drug abuse. *Frontiers in Neuroendocrinology, 29,* 36–47.

Becker, J. B., Prendergast, B. J., & Liang, J. W. (2016). Female rats are not more variable than male rats: A meta-analysis of neuroscience studies. *Biology of Sex Differences, 7,* 34–40.

Bell, H. C., Pellis, S. M., & Kolb, B. (2010). Juvenile peer play experience and the development of the orbitofrontal and medial prefrontal cortex. *Behavioural Brain Research, 207,* 7–13.

Bell, M. R., De Lorme, K. C., Figueira, R. J., Kashy, D. A., & Sisk, C. L. (2013). Adolescent gain in positive valence of a socially relevant stimulus: Engagement of the mesocorticolimbic reward circuitry. *European Journal of Neuroscience, 37,* 457–468.

Bell, M. R., Meerts, S. H., & Sisk, C. L. (2010). Male Syrian hamsters demonstrate a conditioned place preference for sexual behavior and female chemosensory stimuli. *Hormones and Behavior, 58,* 410–414.

Bell, M. R., Meerts, S. H., & Sisk, C. L. (2013). Adolescent brain maturation is necessary for adult-typical mesocorticolimbic responses to a rewarding social cue. *Developmental Neurobiology, 73,* 856–869.

Bell, M. R., & Sisk, C. L. (2013). Dopamine mediates testosterone-induced social reward in male Syrian hamsters. *Endocrinology, 154,* 1225–1234.

Beltz, A. M., & Berenbaum, S. A. (2013). Cognitive effects of variations in pubertal timing: Is puberty a period of brain organization for human sex-typed cognition? *Hormones and Behavior, 63,* 823–828.

Benarroch, E. E. (2013). Oxytocin and vasopressin: Social neuropeptides with complex neuromodulatory functions. *Neurology, 80,* 1521–1528.

Benes, F. M. (1989). Myelination of cortical-hippocampal relays during late adolescence. *Schizophrenia Bulletin, 15,* 585–593.

Benes, F. M., Taylor, J. B., & Cunningham, M. C. (2000). Convergence and plasticity of monoaminergic systems in the medial prefrontal cortex during the postnatal period: Implications for the development of psychopathology. *Cerebral Cortex, 10,* 1014–1027.

Benes, F. M., Turtle, M., Khan, Y., & Farol, P. (1994). Myelination of a key relay zone in the hippocampal formation occurs in the human brain during childhood, adolescence, and adulthood. *Archives of General Psychiatry, 51,* 477–484.

Benes, F. M., Vincent, S. L., Molloy, R., & Khan, Y. (1996). Increased interaction of dopamine-immunoreactive varicosities with GABA neurons of rat medial prefrontal cortex occurs during the postweanling period. *Synapse, 23,* 237–245.

Benowitz, N. L. (2010). Nicotine addiction. *New England Journal of Medicine, 362,* 2295–2303.

Berenbaum, S. A., & Beltz, A. M. (2011). Sexual differentiation of human behavior: Effects of prenatal and pubertal organizational hormones. *Frontiers in Neuroendocrinology, 32,* 183–200.

Bhasin, S., Yuan, Q. X., Steiner, B. S., & Swerdloff, R. S. (1987). Hormonal effects of gonadotropin-releasing hormone (GnRH) agonist in men: Effects of long term treatment with GnRH agonist infusion and androgen. *Journal of Clinical Endocrinology and Metabolism, 65,* 568–574.

Bhatara, V., Feil, M., Hoagwood, K., Vitiello, B., & Zima, B. (2004). National trends in concomitant psychotropic medication with stimulants in pediatric visits: Practice versus knowledge. *Journal of Attention Disorders, 7,* 217–226.

Birrell, J. M., & Brown, V. J. (2000). Medial frontal cortex mediates perceptual attentional set shifting in the rat. *Journal of Neuroscience, 20,* 4320–4324.

Blakemore, S.-J. (2012). Imaging brain development: The adolescent brain. *NeuroImage, 61,* 397–406.

Blakemore, S.-J., Burnett, S., & Dahl, R. E. (2010). The role of puberty in the developing adolescent brain. *Human Brain Mapping, 31,* 926–933.

Blakemore, S.-J., & Choudhury, S. (2006). Development of the adolescent brain: Implications for executive function and social cognition. *Journal of Child Psychology and Psychiatry, 47,* 296–312.

Blizter, R. D., Gil, O., & Landau, E. M. (1990). Long-term potentiation in rat hippocampus is inhibited by low concentrations of ethanol. *Brain Research, 537,* 203–208.

Brand, T., & Slob, A. K. (1988). Peripubertal castration of male rats, adult open field ambulation and partner preference behavior. *Behavioural Brain Research, 30,* 111–117.

Brandon, C. L., Marinelli, M., & White, F. J. (2003). Adolescent exposure to methylphenidate alters the activity of rat midbrain dopamine neurons. *Biological Psychiatry, 54,* 1338–1344.

Brannvall, K., Bogdanovic, N., Korhonen, L., & Lindholm, D. (2005). 19-Nortestosterone influences neural stem cell proliferation and neurogensis in the rat brain. *European Journal of Neuroscience, 21,* 871–878.

Bredewold, R., & Veenema, A. H. (2018). Sex differences in the regulation of social and anxiety-related behaviors: Insights from vassopressin and oxytocin brain systems. *Current Opinions in Neurobiology, 49,* 132–140.

Bredy, T. W., Humpartzoomian, R. A., Cain, D. P., & Meaney, M. J. (2003). Partial reversal of the effect of maternal care on cognitive function through environmental enrichment. *Neuroscience, 118,* 571–576.

Bredy, T. W., Zhang, T. Y., Grant, R. J., Diorio, J., & Meaney, M. J. (2004). Peripubertal environmental enrichment reverses the effects of maternal care on hippocampal development and glutamate receptor subunit expression. *European Journal of Neuroscience, 20,* 1355–1362.

Bridge, J. A., Iyengar, S., Salary, C. B., Barbe, R. P., Birmaher, B., Pincus, H. A., . . . Brent, D. A. (2007). Clinical response and risk for reported suicidal ideation and suicide attempts in pediatric antidepressant treatment: A meta-analysis of randomized controlled trials. *Journal of the American Medical Association, 297,* 1683–1696.

Bridge, J. A., Salary, C. B., Birmaher, B., Asare, A. G., & Brent, D. A. (2005). The risks and benefits of antidepressant treatment for youth depression. *Annals of Medicine, 37,* 404–412.

Broadwater, M. A., Liu, W., Crews, F. T., & Spear, L. P. (2014). Persistent loss of hippocampal neurogenesis and increased cell death following adolescent, but not adult, chronic ethanol exposure. *Developmental Neuroscience, 36,* 297–305.

Brower, K. J. (2002). Anabolic steroid abuse and dependence. *Current Psychiatry Reports, 4,* 377–387.

Bruijnzeel, A. W., Bauzo, R. M., Munikoti, V., Rodrick, G. B., Yamada, H., Fornal, C. A., . . . Jacobs, B. L. (2011). Tobacco smoke diminishes neurogenesis and promotes gliogenesis in the dentate gyrus of adolescent rats. *Brain Research, 1413,* 32–42.

Burnett, S., Sebastian, C., Kadosh, K .C., & Blakemore, S.-J. (2011). The social brain in adolescence: Evidence from functional magnetic resonance imaging and behavioural studies. *Neuroscience and Biobehavioral Reviews, 35,* 1654–1664.

Burton, C. L., & Fletcher, P. J. (2012). Age and sex differences in impulsive action in rats: The role of dopamine and glutamate. *Behavioural Brain Research, 230,* 21–33.

Buynitsky, T., & Mostofsky, D. I. (2009). Restraint stress in biobehavioral research: Recent developments. *Neuroscience and Biobehavioral Reviews, 33,* 1089–1098.

Byne, W., Bradley, S. J., Coleman, E., Eyler, A. E., Green, R., Menvielle, E. J., ... Tompkins, D. A. (2012). Report of the American Psychiatric Association Task Force on treatment of gender identity disorder. *Archives of Sexual Behavior, 41,* 759–796.

Cadete-Leite, A., Alves, M. C., Paula-Barbosa, M. M., Uylings, H. B. M., & Tavares, M. A. (1990). Quantitative analysis of basal dendrites of prefrontal pyramidal cells after chronic alcohol consumption and withdrawal in the adult rat. *Alcohol and Alcoholism, 25,* 467–475.

Cao, J., Belluzzi, J. D., Loughlin, S. E., Dao, J. M., Chen, Y., & Leslie, F. M. (2010). Locomotor and stress responses to nicotine differ in adolescent and adult rats. *Pharmacology, Biochemistry, and Behavior, 96,* 82–90.

Carrillo, M., Ricci, L. A., & Melloni, R. H., Jr. (2009). Adolescent anabolic androgenic steroids reorganize the glutamatergic neural circuitry in the hypothalamus. *Brain Research, 1249,* 118–127.

Casadio, P., Fernandes, C., Murray, R. M., & Di Forti, M. (2011). Cannabis use in young people: The risk for schizophrenia. *Neuroscience and Biobehavioral Reviews, 35,* 1779–1787.

Casey, B. J., Duhoux, S., & Cohen, M. M. (2010). Adolescence: What do transmission, transition, and translation have to do with it? *Neuron, 67,* 749–760.

Casey, B. J., Getz, S., & Galvan, A. (2008). The adolescent brain. *Developmental Review, 28,* 62–77.

Casey, B. J., Giedd, J., & Thomas, K. M. (2000). Structural and functional brain development and its relation to cognitive development. *Biological Psychology, 54,* 241–257.

Casey, B. J., Tottenham, N., Liston, C., & Durston, S. (2005). Imaging the developing brain: What have we learned about cognitive development? *Trends in Cognitive Sciences, 9,* 104–110.

Castellano, J. M., Roa, J., Luque, R. M., Dieguez, C., Aguilar, E., Pinilla, L., & Tena-Sempere, M. (2009). KiSS1/kisspeptins and the metabolic control of reproduction: Physiologic roles and putative physiopathological implications. *Peptides, 30,* 139–145.

Cauffman, E., & Steinberg, L. (2000). (Im)maturity of judgment in adolescence: Why adolescents may be less culpable than adults. *Behavioral Sciences and the Law, 18,* 741–760.

Cavaliere, C., Cirillo, G., Bianco, M. R., Adriani, W., De Simone, A., Leo, D., ... Papa, M. (2012). Methylphenidate administration determines enduring changes in neuro-glial network in rats. *European Neuropharmacology, 22,* 53–63.

Centers for Disease Control. (2010). Increasing prevalence of parent-reported attention-deficit/hyperactivity disorder among children—United States, 2003 and 2007. *Morbidity and Mortality Weekly Report, 59,* 1439–1443.

Cerqueira, J. J., Mailliet, F., Almeida, O. F., Jay, T. M., & Sousa, N. (2007). The prefrontal cortex as a key target of the maladaptive response to stress. *Journal of Neuroscience, 27,* 2781–2787.

Chaker, Z., George, C., Petrovska, M., Caron, J. B., Lacube, J. B., Caille, I., & Holzenberger, M. (2016). Hypothalamic neurogenesis persists in the aging brain and is controlled by energy-sensing IGF-I pathway. *Neurobiology of Aging, 41,* 64–72.

Chandler, L. J. (2003). Ethanol and brain plasticity: Receptors and molecular networks of the postsynaptic density as targets of ethanol. *Pharmacology and Therapeutics, 99,* 311–326.

Chang, L., Yakupov, R., Cloak, C., & Ernst, T. (2006). Marijuana use is associated with a reorganized visual-attention network and cerebellar hypoactivation. *Brain, 129,* 1096–1112.

Chapman, P. F., Ramsay, M. F., Krezel, W., & Knevett, S. G. (2003). Synaptic plasticity in the amygdala comparisons with hippocampus. *Annals of the New York Academy of Sciences, 985,* 114–124.

Chehab, F. F., Mounzih, K., Lu, R., & Lim, M. E. (1997). Early onset of reproductive function in normal female mice treated with leptin. *Science, 275,* 88–90.

Chein, J., Albert, D., O'Brien, L., Uckert, K., & Steinberg, L. (2011). Peers increase adolescent risk taking by enhancing activity in the brain's reward circuitry. *Developmental Science, 14,* F1–F10.

Chevrier, L., Guimiot, F., & de Roux, N. (2011). GnRH receptor mutations in isolated gonadotropic deficiency. *Molecular and Cellular Endocrinology, 346,* 21–28.

Chin, V. S., Van Skike, C. E., & Matthews, D. B. (2010). Effects of ethanol on hippocampal function during adolescence: A look at the past and thoughts on the future. *Alcohol, 44,* 3–14.

Christensen, L. W., Nance, D. M., & Gorski, R. A. (1977). Effects of hypothalamic and preoptic lesions on reproductive behavior in male rats. *Brain Research Bulletin, 2,* 137–141.

Cicchetti, D., & Toth, S. L. (1998). The development of depression in children and adolescents. *American Psychologist, 53,* 221–241.

Clark, A. S., & Henderson, L. P. (2003). Behavioral and physiological responses to anabolic-androgenic steroids. *Neuroscience and Biobehavioral Reviews, 27,* 413–436.

Clarke, I. J., & Cummins, J. T. (1982). The temporal relationship between gonadotropin releasing hormone (GnRH) and luteinizing hormone (LH) secretion in ovariectomized ewes. *Endocrinology, 111,* 1737–1739.

Clarkson, J., Boon, W. C., Simpson, E. R., & Herbison, A. E. (2009). Postnatal development of an estradiol-kisspeptin feedback mechanism implicated in puberty onset. *Endocrinology, 150,* 3214–3220.

Clarkson, J., Han, S.-K., Liu, X., Lee, K., & Herbison, A. E. (2010). Neurobiological mechanisms underlying kisspeptin activation of gonadotropin-releasing hormone (GnRH) neurons at puberty. *Molecular and Cellular Endocrinology, 324,* 45–50.

Clarkson, J., & Herbison, A. E. (2006). Development of GABA and glutamate signaling at the GnRH neuron in relation to puberty. *Molecular and Cellular Endocrinology, 254–255,* 32–38.

Conger, J., & Petersen, A. (1984). *Adolescence and youth: Psychological development in a changing world.* New York, NY: Harper and Row.

Conrad, C. D., Galea, L. A., Kuroda, Y., & McEwen, B. S. (1996). Chronic stress impairs rat spatial memory on the Y maze, and this effect is blocked by tianeptine pretreatment. *Behavioral Neuroscience, 110,* 1321–1334.

Conrad, C. D., Magarinos, A. M., LeDoux, J. E., & McEwen, B. S. (1999). Repeated restraint stress facilitates fear conditioning independently of causing hippocampal CA3 dendritic atrophy. *Behavioral Neuroscience, 113,* 902–913.

Cooke, B., Hegstrom, C. D., Villeneuve, L. S., & Breedlove, S. M. (1998). Sexual differentiation of the vertebrate brain: Principles and mechanisms. *Frontiers in Neuroendocrinology, 19,* 323–362.

Corbier, P., Kerdelhue, B., Picon, R., & Roffi, J. (1978). Changes in testicular weight and serum gonadotropin and testosterone levels before, during, and after birth in the perinatal rat. *Endocrinology, 103,* 1985–1991.

Costello, E. J., Mustillo, S., Erkanli, A., Keeler, G., & Angold, A. (2003). Prevalence and development of psychiatric disorders in childhood and adolescence. *Archives of General Psychiatry, 60,* 837–844.

Cote, J. E. (2014). The dangerous myth of emerging adulthood: An evidence-based critique of a flawed developmental theory. *Applied Developmental Science, 18,* 177–188.

Cowen, D. S., Takase, L. F., Fornal, C. A., & Jacobs, B. L. (2008). Age-dependent decline in hippocampal neurogenesis is not altered by chronic treatment with fluoxetine. *Brain Research, 1228,* 14–19.

Cressman, V. L., Balaban, J., Steinfeld, S., Shemyakin, A., Graham, P., Parisot, N., & Moore, H. (2010). Prefrontal cortical inputs to the basal amygdala undergo pruning during late adolescence in the rat. *Journal of Comparative Neurology, 518,* 2693–2709.

Crews, F. T., Braun, C. J., Hoplight, B., Switzer, R. C., & Knapp, D. J. (2000). Binge ethanol consumption causes differential brain damage in young adolescent rats compared with adult rats. *Alcoholism: Clinical and Experimental Research, 24,* 1712–1723.

Crews, F. T., He, J., & Hodge, C. (2007). Adolescent cortical development: A critical period of vulnerability for addiction. *Pharmacology, Biochemistry, and Behavior, 86,* 189–199.

Crews, F. T., Mdzinarishvili, A., Kim, D., He, J., & Nixon, K. (2006). Neurogenesis in adolescent brain is potently inhibited by ethanol. *Neuroscience, 137,* 437–445.

Cuffe, S. P., McKeown, R. E., Jackson, K. J., Addy, C. L., Abramson, R., & Garrison, C. Z. (2001). Prevalence of attention-deficit/hyperactivity disorder in a community sample of older adolescents. *Journal of the American Academy of Child and Adolescent Psychiatry, 40,* 1037–1044.

Cunningham, M. G., Bhattacharyya, S., & Benes, F. M. (2002). Amygdalo-cortical sprouting continues into early adulthood: Implications for the development of normal and abnormal function during adolescence. *Journal of Comparative Neurology, 453,* 116–130.

Cunningham, M. J., Clifton, D. K., & Steiner, R. A. (1999). Leptin's actions on the reproductive axis: Perspectives and mechanisms. *Biology of Reproduction, 60,* 216–222.

Cunningham, R. L., Claiborne, B. J., & McGinnis, M. Y. (2007). Pubertal exposure to anabolic androgenic steroids increases spine densities on neurons in the limbic system of male rats. *Neuroscience, 150,* 609–615.

Dahl, R. E. (2004). Adolescent brain development: A period of vulnerabilities and opportunities. *Annals of the New York Academy of Sciences, 1021,* 1–22.

Dahl, R. E., & Gunnar, M. R. (2009). Heightened stress responsiveness and emotional reactivity during pubertal maturation: Implications for psychopathology. *Development and Psychopathology, 21,* 1–6.

Dalley, J. W., Cardinal, R. N., & Robbins, T. W. (2004). Prefrontal executive and cognitive functions in rodents: Neural and neurochemical substrates. *Neuroscience and Biobehavioral Reviews, 28,* 771–784.

Damasio, H., Grabowski, T., Frank, R., Galaburda, A. M., & Damasio, A. R. (1994). The return of Phineas Gage: Clues about the brain from the skull of a famous patient. *Science, 264,* 1102–1105.

David, J. T., Cervantes, M. C., Trosky, K. A., Salinas, J. A., & Delville, Y. (2004). A neural network underlying individual differences in emotion and aggression in male golden hamsters. *Neuroscience, 126,* 567–578.

De Bellis, M. D., Clark, D. B., Beers, S. R., Soloff, P. H., Boring, A. M., Hall, J. J., ... Keshavan, M .S. (2000). Hippocampal volume in adolescent-onset alcohol use disorder. American Journal of Psychiatry 157, 737–744.

De Bellis, M. D., Keshavan, M., Beers, S. R., Hall, J., Frustaci, K., Masalehdan, A., ... Boring, A. M. (2001). Sex differences in brain maturation during childhood and adolescence. *Cerebral Cortex, 11,* 552–557.

De Bond, J.-A.P., & Smith, J. T. (2014). Kisspeptin and energy balance in reproduction. *Reproduction, 147,* R53–R63.

de Fonseca, F. R., del Arco, I., Bermudez-Silva, F. J., Bilbao, A., Cippitelli, A., & Navarro, M. (2004). The endocannabinoid system: Physiology and pharmacology. *Alcohol and Alcoholism, 40,* 2–14.

de Kloet, E. R., Joels, M., & Holsboer, F. (2005). Stress and the brain: From adaptation to disease. *Nature Reviews Neuroscience, 6,* 463–475.

de Kloet, E. R., Oitzl, M. S., & Joels, M. (1999). Stress and cognition: Are corticosteroids good or bad guys? *Trends in Neurosciences, 22,* 422–426.

de Kloet, E. R., Vreugdenhil, E., Oitzl, M. S., & Joels, M. (1998). Brain corticosteroid receptor balance in health and disease. *Endocrine Reviews, 19,* 269–301.

de la Pena, J. B., Ahsan, H. M., Botanas, C. J., dela Pena, I. J., Woo, T., Kim, H. J., & Cheong, J. H. (2016). Cigarette smoke exposure during adolescence but not adulthood induces anxiety-like behavior and locomotor stimulation in rats during withdrawal. *International Journal of Developmental Neuroscience, 55,* 49–55.

De Lorme, K. C., Bell, M. R., & Sisk, C. L. (2012). Maturation of social reward in adult male Syrian hamsters does not depend on organizational effects of pubertal testosterone. *Hormones and Behavior, 62,* 180–185.

De Lorme, K. C., & Sisk, C. L. (2013). Pubertal testosterone programs context-appropriate agonistic behavior and associated neural activation patterns in male Syrian hamsters. *Physiology and Behavior, 112,* 1–7.

De Lorme, K. C., & Sisk, C. L. (2016). The organizational effects of pubertal testosterone on sexual proficiency in adult male Syrian hamsters. *Physiology and Behavior, 165,* 273–277.

de Roux, N., Genin, E., Carel, J.-C., Matsuda, F., Chaussain, J.-L., & Milgrom, E. (2003). Hypogonadotropic hypogonadism due to loss of function of the KiSS1-dervied peptide receptor GRP54. *Proceedings of the National Academy of Sciences, 100,* 10972–10976.

Dekaban, A. S., & Sadowsky, D. (1978). Changes in brain weights during the span of human life: Relation of brain weight to body heights and body weight. *Annals of Neurology, 4,* 345–356.

DeLeon, K. R., Grimes, J. M., & Melloni, R. H., Jr. (2002). Repeated anabolic-androgenic steroid treatment during adolescence increases vasopressin V1a receptor binding in Syrian hamsters: Correlation with offensive aggression. *Hormones and Behavior, 42,* 182–191.

Dennsion, M., Whittle, S., Yucel, M., Vijayakumar, N., Kline, A., Simmons, J., & Allen, N. B. (2013). Mapping subcortical brain maturation during adolescence: Evidence of hemisphere- and sex-specific longitudinal changes. *Developmental Science, 16,* 772–791.

Dickerson, S. M., & Gore, A. C. (2007). Estrogenic environmental endocrine-disrupting chemical effects on reproductive neuroendocrine function and dysfunction across the life cycle. *Reviews in Endocrinology and Metabolic Disorders, 8,* 143–159.

Dimler, L. M., & Natsuaki, M. N. (2015). The effects of pubertal timing on externalizing behaviors in adolescence and early adulthood: A meta-analytic review. *Journal of Adolescence, 45,* 160–170.

Dodge, K. A. (1993). Social-cognitive mechanisms in the development of conduct disorder and depression. *Annual Review of Psychology, 44,* 559–584.

Donaldson, Z. R., & Young, L. J. (2008). Oxytocin, vasopressin, and the neurogenetics of sociality. *Science, 322,* 900–904.

Doremus, T. L., Brunell, S. C., Varlinskaya, E. I., & Spear, L. P. (2003). Anxiogenic effects during withdrawal from acute ethanol in adolescent and adult rats. *Pharmacology, Biochemistry and Behavior, 75,* 411–418.

Doremus-Fitzwater, T. L., Barreto, M., & Spear, L. P. (2012). Age-related differences in impulsivity among adolescent and adult Sprague–Dawley rats. *Behavioral Neuroscience, 126,* 735–741.

Doremus-Fitzwater, T. L., & Spear, L. P. (2016). Reward-centricity and attenuated aversions: An adolescent phenotype emerging from studies in laboratory animals. *Neuroscience and Biobehavioral Reviews, 70,* 121–134.

Doremus-Fitzwater, T. L., Varlinskaya, E. I., & Spear, L. P. (2010). Motivational systems in adolescence: Possible implications for age differences in substance abuse and other risk-taking behaviors. *Brain and Cognition, 72,* 114–123.

Doura, M. B., Luu, T. V., Lee, N. H., & Perry, D. C. (2010). Persistent gene expression changes in ventral tegmental area of adolescent but not adult rats in response to chronic nicotine. *Neuroscience, 170,* 503–513.

Dranovsky, A., & Hen, R. (2006). Hippocampal neurogenesis: Regulation by stress and antidepressants. *Biological Psychiatry, 59,* 1136–1143.

Drysdale, A. J., & Platt, B. (2003). Cannabinoids: Mechanisms and therapeutic applications in the CNS. *Current Medicinal Chemistry, 10,* 2719–2732.

Dwyer, A. A., Quinton, R., Pitteloud, N., & Morin, D. (2015). Psychosexual development in men with congenital hypogonadotropic hypogonadism on long-term treatment: A mixed methods study. *Sexual Medicine, 3,* 32–41.

Eiland, L., Ramroop, J., Hill, M. N., Manely, J., & McEwen, B. S. (2012). Chronic juvenile stress produces corticolimbic dendritic architectural remodeling and modulates emotional behavior in male and female rats. *Psychoneuroendocrinology, 37,* 39–47.

Eiland, L., & Romeo, R. D. (2013). Stress and the developing adolescent brain. *Neuroscience, 249,* 162–171.

Elenkov, I., Kovacs, K., Kiss, J., Bertok, L., & Vizi, E. S. (1992). Lipopolysaccharide is able to bypass corticotropin-releasing factor in affecting plasma ACTH and corticosterone levels: Evidence from rats with lesions of the paraventricular nucleus. *Journal of Endocrinology, 133,* 231–236.

Ellgren, M., Artmann, A., Tkalych, O., Gupta, A., Hansen, H. S., Hansen, S. H., . . . Hurd, Y. L. (2008). Dynamic changes of the endogenous cannabinoid and opioid mesocorticolimbic systems during adolescence: THC effects. *European Neuropsychopharmacology, 18,* 826–834.

Ernst, M., & Fudge, J. L. (2009). A developmental neurobiological model of motivated behavior: Anatomy, connectivity and ontogeny of the triadic nodes. *Neuroscience and Biobehavioral Reviews, 33,* 367–382.

Ernst, M., Nelson, E. E., Jazbec, S., McClure, E. B., Monk, C. S., Leibenluft, E., . . . Pine, D. S. (2005). Amygdala and nucleus accumbens in responses to receipt and omission of gains in adults and adolescents. *NeuroImage, 25,* 1279–1291.

Ernst, M., Pine, D. S., & Hardin, M. (2006). Triadic model of the neurobiology of motivated behavior in adolescence. *Psychological Medicine, 36,* 299–312.

Evans, A. C., & the Brain Development Cooperative Group. (2006). The NIH MRI study of normal brain development. *NeuroImage, 30,* 184–202.

Farrell, S. F., & McGinnis, M. Y. (2004). Long-term effects of pubertal anabolic-androgenic steroid exposure on reproductive and aggressive behaviors in male rats. *Hormones and Behavior, 46,* 193–203.

Feinberg, I. (1982). Schizophrenia: Caused by a fault in programmed synaptic elimination during adolescence? *Journal of Psychiatric Research, 17,* 319–334.

Fendt, M., & Fanselow, M. S. (1999). The neuroanatomical and neurochemical basis of conditioned fear. *Neuroscience and Biobehavioral Reviews, 23,* 743–760.

Ferris, C. F., Axelson, J. F., Shinto, L. H., & Albers, H. E. (1987). Scent marking and the maintenance of dominant/subordinate status in male golden hamsters. *Physiology and Behavior, 40,* 661–664.

Ferris, C. F., Gold, L., De Vries, G. J., & Potegal, M. (1990). Evidence for a functional and anatomical relationship between the lateral septum and the hypothalamus in the control of flank marking behavior in golden hamsters. *Journal of Comparative Neurology, 293,* 476–485.

Fiala, J. C., Spacek, J., & Harris, K. M. (2002). Dendritic spine pathology: Cause or consequence of neurological disorders? *Brain Research Reviews, 39,* 29–54.

Field, E. F., Whishaw, I. Q., Forgie, M. L., & Pellis, S. M. (2004). Neonatal and pubertal, but not adult, ovarian steroids are necessary for the development of female-typical patterns of dodging to protect a food item. *Behavioral Neuroscience, 118,* 1293–1304.

Forbes, C. E., & Grafman, J. (2010). The role of the human prefrontal cortex in social cognition and moral judgement. *Annual Review of Neuroscience, 33,* 299–324.

Forger, N. G. (2006). Cell death and sexual differentiation of the nervous system. *Neuroscience, 138,* 929–938.

Fowler, C. D., Liu, Y., Ouimet, C., & Wang, Z. (2002). The effects of social environment on adult neurogenesis in the female prairie vole. *Journal of Neurobiology, 51,* 115–128.

Fox, C., Merali, Z., & Harrison, C. (2006). Therapeutic and protective effects of environmental enrichment against psychogenic and neurogenic stress. *Behavioural Brain Research, 175,* 1–8.

Francis, D. D., Diorio, J., Plotsky, P. M., & Meaney, M. J. (2002). Environmental enrichment reverses the effects of maternal separation on stress reactivity. *Journal of Neuroscience, 22,* 7840–7843.

Frederick, A. L., & Stanwood, G. D. (2009). Drugs, biogenic amine targets and the developing brain. *Developmental Neuroscience, 31,* 7–22.

Friedman, J. (2016). The long road to leptin. *Journal of Clinical Investigation, 126,* 4727–4734.

Frisch, R. E., & Revelle, R. (1970). Height and weight at menarche and a hypothesis of critical body weights and adolescent events. *Science, 169,* 397–399.

Galvan, A. (2010). Adolescent development of the reward system. *Frontiers in Human Neuroscience, 4,* 6.

Galvan, A., Hare, T. A., Parra, C. E., Penn, J., Voss, H., Glover, G., & Casey, B. J. (2006). Earlier development of the accumbens relative to orbitofrontal cortex might underlie risk-taking behavior in adolescents. *Journal of Neuroscience, 26,* 6885–6892.

Galvan, A., & McGlennen, K. M. (2012). Daily stress increases risky decision-making in adolescents: A preliminary study. *Developmental Psychobiology, 54,* 433–440.

Galvao, T. F., Silva, M. T., Zimmermann, I. R., Souza, K. M., Martins, S. S., & Pereira, M. G. (2014). Pubertal timing in girls and depression: A systematic review. *Journal of Affective Disorders, 155,* 13–19.

Gaoni, Y., & Mechoulam, R. (1964). Isolation, structure, and partial synthesis of an active constituent of hashish. *Journal of the American Chemical Society, 86,* 1646–1647.

Gardner, M., & Steinberg, L. (2005). Peer influence on risk taking, risk preference, and risky decision in making adolescence and adulthood: An experimental study. *Developmental Psychology, 41,* 625–635.

Gaspar, P., Cases, O., & Maroteaux, L. (2003). The developmental role of serotonin: News from mouse molecular genetics. *Nature Reviews Neuroscience, 4,* 1002–1012.

Ge, X., Natsuaki, M. N., Neiderhiser, J. M., & Reiss, D. (2009). The longitudinal effects of stressful life events on adolescent depression are buffered by parent–child closeness. *Development and Psychopathology, 21,* 621–635.

Geier, C. F., Terwilliger, R., Teslovich, T., Velanova, K., & Luna, B. (2010). Immaturities in reward processing and its influence on inhibitory control in adolescence. *Cerebral Cortex, 20,* 1613–1629.

Gest, S. D., Reed, M.-G. J., & Masten, A. S. (1999). Measuring developmental changes in exposure to adversity: A life chart and rating scale approach. *Development and Psychopathology, 11,* 171–192.

Gianaros, P. J., Jennings, J. R., Sheu, L. K., Greer, P. J., Kuller, L. H., & Matthews, K. A. (2007). Prospective reports of chronic life stress predict decreased grey matter volume in the hippocampus. *NeuroImage, 35,* 795–803.

Gibbons, R. D., Brown, C. H., Hur, K., Marcus, S. M., Bhaumik, D. K., Erkens, J. A., . . . Mann, J. J. (2007). Early evidence on the effects of regulators' suicidality warnings on SSRI prescriptions and suicide in children and adolescents. *American Journal of Psychiatry, 164,* 1356–1363.

Giedd, J. N. (2004). Structural magnetic resonance imaging of the adolescent brain. *Annals of the New York Academy of Sciences, 1021,* 77–85.

Giedd, J. N. (2008). The teen brain: Insights from neuroimaging. *Journal of Adolescent Health, 42,* 335–343.

Giedd, J. N., Blumenthal, J., Jeffries, N. O., Castellanos, F. X., Liu, H., Zijdenbos, A., . . . Rapoport, J. L. (1999). Brain development during childhood and adolescence: A longitudinal MRI study. *Nature Neuroscience, 2,* 861–863.

Giedd, J. N., Clasen, L. S., Lenroot, R., Greenstein, D., Wallace, G. L., Ordaz, S., . . . Chrousos, G. P. (2006). Puberty-related influences on brain development. *Molecular and Cellular Endocrinology, 254–255,* 154–162.

Giedd, J. N., & Rapoport, J. L. (2010). Structural MRI of pediatric brain development: What have we learned and where are we going? *Neuron, 67,* 728–734.

Giedd, J. N., Raznahan, A., Alexander-Bloch, A., Schmitt, E., Gogtay, N., & Rapoport, J. L. (2015). Child psychiatry branch of the National Institute of Mental Health longitudinal structural magnetic resonance imaging study of human brain development. *Neuropsychopharmacology, 40,* 43–49.

Giedd, J. N., Snell, J. W., Lange, N., Rajapakse, J. C., Casey, B. J., Kozuch, P. L., . . . Rapoport, J. L. (1996). Quantitative magnetic resonance imaging of human brain development: Ages 4–18. *Cerebral Cortex, 6,* 551–560.

Giedd, J. N., Vaituzis, A. C., Hamburger, S. D., Lange, N., Rajapakse, J. C., Kaysen, D., . . . Rapoport, J. L. (1996). Quantitative MRI of the temporal lobe, amygdala, and hippocampus in normal human development: Ages 4–18 years. *Journal of Comparative Neurology, 366,* 223–230.

Gluckman, P. D., & Hanson, M. A. (2006a). Changing times: The evolution of puberty. *Molecular and Cellular Endocrinology, 254–255,* 26–31.

Gluckman, P. D., & Hanson, M. A. (2006b). Evolution, development and timing of puberty. *Trends in Endocrinology and Metabolism, 17,* 7–12.

Goble, K. H., Bain, Z. A., Padow, V. A., Lui, P., Klein, Z. A., & Romeo, R. D. (2011). Pubertal-related changes in hypothalamic-pituitary-adrenal axis reactivity and cytokine secretion in response to an immunological stressor. *Journal of Neuroendocrinology, 23,* 129–135.

Goddings, A.-L., Heyes, S. B., Bird, G., Viner, R. M., & Blakemore, S.-J. (2012). The relationship between puberty and social emotion processing. *Developmental Science, 15,* 801–811.

Goddings, A.-L., Mills, K. L., Clasen, L. S., Giedd, J. N., Viner, R. M., & Blakemore, S.-J. (2014). The influence of puberty on subcortical brain development. *NeuroImage, 88,* 242–251.

Gogtay, N., Giedd, J. N., Lusk, L., Hayashi, K. M., Greenstein, D., Vaituzis, A. C., . . . Thompson, P. M. (2004). Dynamic mapping of human cortical development during childhood through early adulthood. *Proceedings of the National Academy of Sciences, 101,* 8174–8179.

Goldenberg, D., & Galvan, A. (2015). The use of functional and effective connectivity techniques to understand the developing brain. *Developmental Cognitive Neuroscience, 12,* 155–164.

Goldman-Rakic, P. S. (1996). The prefrontal landscape: Implications of functional architecture for understanding human mentation and the central executive. *Philosophical Transactions of the Royal Society of London B, 351,* 1445–1453.

Golub, M .S., Collman, G. W., Foster, P. M. D., Kimmel, C. A., Rajpert-De Meyts, E., Reiter, E. O., . . . Toppari, J. (2008). Public health implications of altered puberty timing. *Pediatrics, 121,* S218–S230.

Goodman, R. L., & Lehman, M. N. (2012). Kisspeptin neurons from mice to men: Similarities and differences. *Endocrinology, 153,* 5105–5118.

Goodnick, P. J., & Goldstein, B. J. (1998). Selective serotonin reuptake inhibitors in affective disorders I. Basic pharmacology. *Journal of Psychopharmacology, 12,* S5–S20.

Gould, E. (2007). How widespread is adult neurogenesis in mammals. *Nature Reviews Neuroscience, 8,* 481–488.

Gould, E., McEwen, B. S., Tanapat, P., Galea, L. A., & Fuchs, E. (1997). Neurogenesis in the dentate gyrus of the adult tree shrew is regulated by psychosocial stress and NMDA receptor activation. *Journal of Neuroscience, 17,* 2492–2498.

Graber, J. A. (2013). Pubertal timing and the development of psychopathology in adolescence and beyond. *Hormones and Behavior, 64,* 262–269.

Grant, A., Hoops, D., Labelle-Dumais, C., Prevost, M., Rajabi, H., Kolb, B., . . . Flores, C. (2007). Netrin-1 receptor-deficient mice show enhanced mesocortical dopamine transmission and blunted behavioural responses to amphetamine. *European Journal of Neuroscience, 26,* 3215–3228.

Grant, B. F., & Dawson, D. A. (1997). Age at onset of alcohol use and its association with DSM-IV alcohol abuse and dependence: Results from the national longitudinal alcohol epidemiologic survey. *Journal of Substance Abuse, 9,* 103–110.

Grant, K. E., Compas, B. E., Stuchlmacher, A. F., Thurn, A. E., McMahon, S. D., & Halpert, J. A. (2003). Stressors and child and adolescent psychopathology: Moving from markers to mechanisms of risk. *Psychological Bulletin, 129,* 447–466.

Grant, K. E., Compas, B. E., Thurm, A. E., McMahon, S. D., & Gipson, P. Y. (2004). Stressors and child and adolescent psychopathology: Measurement issues and prospective effects. *Journal of Clinical Child and Adolescent Psychology, 33,* 412–425.

Gray, J. D., Punsoni, M., Tabori, N. E., Melton, J. T., Fanslow, V., Ward, M. J., . . . Milner, T. A. (2007). Methylphenidate administration to juvenile rats alters brain areas involved in cognition, motivated behaviors, appetite, and stress. *Journal of Neuroscience, 27,* 7196–7207.

Greely, H., Sahakian, B., Harris, J., Kessler, R. C., Gazzaniga, M., Campbell, P., Farah, & M. J. (2008). Towards responsible use of cognitive-enhancing drugs by the healthy. *Nature, 456,* 702–705.

Greenough, W. T., Black, J. E., & Wallace, C. S. (1987). Experience and brain development. *Child Development, 58,* 539–559.

Grimes, J. M., & Melloni, R. H., Jr. (2002). Serotonin modulates offensive attack in adolescent anabolic steroid-treated hamsters. *Pharmacology, Biochemistry and Behavior, 73,* 713–721.

Grimes, J. M., & Melloni, R. H., Jr. (2005). Serotonin-1B receptor activity and expression modulate the aggression-stimulating effects of adolescent anabolic steroid exposure in hamsters. *Behavioral Neuroscience, 119,* 1184–1194.

Grimes, J. M., & Melloni, R. H., Jr. (2006). Prolonged alterations in the serotonin neural system following the cessation of adolescent anabolic-androgenic steroid exposure in hamsters (*Mesocricetus auratus*). *Behavioral Neuroscience, 120,* 1242–1251.

Grimes, J. M., Ricci, L. A., & Melloni, R. H., Jr. (2003). Glutamic acid decarboxylase (GAD65) immunoreactivity in brains of aggressive, adolescent anabolic steroid-treated hamsters. *Hormones and Behavior, 44,* 271–280.

Grimes, J. M., Ricci, L. A., & Melloni, R. H., Jr. (2006). Plasticity in anterior hypothalamic vasopressin correlates with aggression during anabolic-androgenic steroid withdrawal in hamsters. *Behavioral Neuroscience, 120,* 115–124.

Guerri, C. (2002). Mechanisms involved in central nervous system dysfunctions induced by prenatal ethanol exposure. *Neurotoxicity Research, 4,* 327–335.

Guillamon, A., de Blas, M. R., & Segovia, S. (1988). Effects of sex steroids on the development of the locus coeruleus in the rat. *Brain Research, 468,* 306–310.

Gunnar, M. R., Wewerka, S., Frenn, K., Long, J. D., & Griggs, C. (2009). Developmental changes in hypothalamus–pituitary–adrenal activity over the transition to adolescence: Normative changes and associations with puberty. *Development and Psychopathology, 21,* 69–85.

Gurley, R. J., Aranow, R., & Katz, M. (1998). Medicinal marijuana: A comprehensive review. *Journal of Psychoactive Drugs, 30,* 137–147.

Hahn, A. C., & Perrett, D. I. (2014). Neural and behavioral responses to attractiveness in adult and infant faces. *Neuroscience and Biobehavioral Reviews, 46,* 591–603.

Hall, G. S. (1904). *Adolescence its psychology and its relations to physiology, anthropology, sociology, sex, crime, religion and education.* New York, NY: D. Appleton.

Hall, R. C. W., Hall, R. C. W., & Chapman, M. J. (2005). Psychiatric complications of anabolic steroid abuse. *Psychosomatics, 46,* 285–290.

Hammad, T. A., Laughren, T., & Racoosin, J. (2006). Suicidality in pediatric patients treated with antidepressant drugs. *Archives of General Psychiatry, 63,* 332–339.

Hampson, E. (1995). Spatial cognition in humans: Possible modulation by androgens and estrogens. *Journal of Psychiatric & Neuroscience, 20,* 397–404.

Han, S.-K., Abraham, I. M., & Herbison, A. E. (2002). Effect of GABA on GnRH neurons switches from depolarization to hyperpolarization at puberty in the female mouse. *Endocrinology, 143,* 1459–1466.

Han, S.-K., Gottsch, M. L., Lee, K. J., Popa, S. M., Smith, J. T., Jakawich, S. K., . . . Herbison, A. E. (2005). Activation of gonadotropin-releasing hormone neurons by kisspeptin as a neuroendocrine switch for the onset of puberty. *Journal of Neuroscience, 25,* 11349–11356.

Harte, L. C., & Dow-Edwards, D. (2010). Sexually dimorphic alterations in locomotion and reversal learning after adolescent tetrahydrocannabinol exposure in the rat. *Neurotoxicology and Teratology, 32,* 515–524.

He, J., & Crews, F. T. (2007). Neurogenesis decreases during brain maturation from adolescence to adulthood. *Pharmacology, Biochemistry, and Behavior, 86,* 327–333.

Hebbard, P. C., King, R. R., Malsbury, C. W., & Harley, C. W. (2003). Two organizational effects of pubertal testosterone in male rats: Transient memory and a shift away from long-term potentiation following a tetanus in hippocampal CA1. *Experimental Neurology, 182,* 470–475.

Hechtman, L., & Greenfield, B. (2003). Long-term use of stimulants in children with attention deficit hyperactivity disorder: Safety, efficacy, and long-term outcome. *Pediatric Drugs, 5,* 787–794.

Heine, V. M., Maslam, S., Joels, M., & Lucassen, P. J. (2004). Prominent decline of newborn cell proliferation, differentiation, and apoptosis in the aging dentate gyrus, in absence of an age-related hypothalamic–pituitary–adrenal axis activation. *Neurobiology of Aging, 25,* 361–375.

Heine, V. M., Maslam, S., Zareno, J., Joels, M., & Lucassen, P. J. (2004). Suppressed proliferation and apoptotic changes in the rat dentate gyrus after acute and chronic stress are reversible. *European Journal of Neuroscience, 19,* 131–144.

Hembree, W. C., Cohen-Kettenis, P. T., Gooren, L., Hannema, S. E., Meyer, W. J., Murad, M. H., . . . Sjoen, G. (2017). Endocrine treatment of gender-dysphoric/gender-incongruent persons: An endocrine society clinical practice guideline. *Journal of Clinical Endocrinology and Metabolism, 102,* 1–35.

Hensch, T. K. (2005). Critical period mechanisms in developing visual cortex. *Current Topics in Developmental Biology, 69,* 215–237.

Herkenham, M., Lynn, A. B., Johnson, M. R., Melvin, L. S., de Costa, B. R., & Rice, K. C. (1991). Characterization and localization of cannabinoid receptors in rat brain: A quantitative in vitro autoradiographic study. *Journal of Neuroscience, 11,* 563–583.

Herkenham, M., Lynn, A. B., Little, M. D., Johnson, M. R., Melvin, L. S., De Costa, B. R., & Rice, K. C. (1989). Cannabinoid receptor localization in brain. *Proceedings of the National Academy of Sciences, 87,* 1932–1936.

Herman-Giddens, M. E., Slora, E. J., Wasserman, R. C., Bourdony, C. J., Bhapkar, M. V., Koch, G. G., & Hasemeier, C. M. (1997). Secondary sexual characteristics and menses in young girls seen in office practice: A study from the Pediatric Research in Office Setting Network. *Pediatrics, 99,* 505–512.

Herman, J. P., Figueiredo, H., Mueller, N. K., Ulrich-Lai, Y., Ostander, M. M., Choi, D. C., & Cullinan, W. E. (2003). Central mechanisms of stress integration: Hierarchical circuitry controlling hypothalamic–pituitary–adrenocortical responsiveness. *Frontiers of Neuroendocrinology, 24,* 151–180.

Herting, M. M., Gautam, P., Spielberg, J. M., Dahl, R. E., & Sowell, E. R. (2015). A longitudinal study: Changes in cortical thickness and surface area during pubertal maturation. *PLOS ONE, 10,* e0119774.

Herting, M. M., Gautam, P., Spielberg, J. M., Kan, E., Dahl, R. E., & Sowell, E. R. (2014). The role of testosterone and estradiol in brain volume changes across adolescence: A longitudinal structural MRI study. *Human Brain Mapping, 35,* 5633–5645.

Herting, M. M., Kim, R., Uban, K. A., Kan, E., Binley, A., & Sowell, E. R. (2017). Longitudinal changes in pubertal maturation and white matter microstructure. *Psychoneuroendocrinology, 81,* 70–79.

Herting, M. M., & Sowell, E. R. (2017). Puberty and structural brain development in humans. *Frontiers in Neuroendocrinology, 44,* 122–137.

Heyser, C. J., Pelletier, M., & Ferris, J. S. (2004). The effects of methylphenidate on novel object exploration in weanling and periadolescent rats. *Annals of the New York Academy of Sciences, 1021,* 465–469.

Hier, D. B., & Crowley, W. F. (1982). Spatial ability in androgen-deficient men. *New England Journal of Medicine, 306,* 1202–1205.

Ho, A., Villacis, A. J., Svirsky, S .E., Foilb, A. R., & Romeo, R. D. (2012). The pubertal-related decline in cellular proliferation and neurogenesis in the dentate gyrus of male rats is independent of the pubertal rise in gonadal hormones. *Developmental Neurobiology, 72,* 743–752.

Hodes, G. E., Yang, L., van Kooy, J., Santollo, J., & Shors, T. J. (2009). Prozac during puberty: Distinctive effects on neurogenesis as a function of age and sex. *Neuroscience, 163,* 609–617.

Hoffman, A. R., & Crowley, W. F. (1982). Induction of puberty in men by long-term pulsatile administration of low-dose gonadotropin-releasing hormone. *New England Journal of Medicine, 307,* 1237–1241.

Holmes, A., & Wellman, C. L. (2009). Stress-induced prefrontal reorganization and executive dysfunction in rodents. *Neuroscience and Biobehavioral Reviews, 33,* 773–783.

Homberg, J. R., Olivier, J. D. A., Blom, T., Arensten, T., van Brunschot, C., Schipper, P., . . . Reneman, L. (2011). Fluoxetine exerts age-dependent effects on behavior and amygdala neuroplasticity in the rat. *PLOS ONE, 6,* e16646.

Hoops, D., & Flores, C. (2017). Making dopamine connections in adolescence. *Trends in Neurosciences, 40,* 709–719.

Hough, C., Bellingham, M., Haraldsen, I. R., McLaughlin, M., Rennie, M., Robinson, J. E., . . . Evans, N. P. (2017). Spatial memory is impaired by peripubertal GnRH agonist treatment and testosterone replacement in sheep. *Psychoneuroendocrinology, 75,* 173–182.

Hough, D., Bellingham, M., Haraldsen, I. R., McLaughlin, M., Robinson, J. E., Solbakk, A. K., & Evans, N. P. (2017). A reduction in long-term spatial memory persists after discontinuation of peripubertal GnRH agonist treatment in sheep. *Psychoneuroendocrinology, 77,* 1–8.

Huey, E. D., Lee, S., Brickman, A. M., Manoochehri, M., Griffith, E., Devanand, D. P., . . . Grafman, J. (2015). Neuropsychiatric effects of neurodegeneration of the medial versus lateral ventral prefrontal cortex in humans. *Cortex, 73,* 1–9.

Huttenlocher, P. R. (1979). Synaptic density in human frontal cortex developmental changes and effects of aging. *Brain Research, 163,* 195–205.

Huttenlocher, P. R., & Dabholkar, A. S. (1997). Regional differences in synaptogenesis in human cerebral cortex. *Journal of Comparative Neurology, 387,* 167–178.

Hyman, S. E. (2003). Methylphenidate-induced plasticity: What should we be looking for? *Biological Psychiatry, 54,* 1310–1311.

Iniguez, S. D., Warren, B. L., Parise, E. M., Alcantara, L. F., Schuh, B., Maffeo, M. L., . . . Bolanos-Guzman, C. A. (2009). Nicotine exposure during adolescence induces a depression-like state in adulthood. *Neuropsychopharmacology, 34,* 1609–1624.

Irvin, R. W., Szot, P., Dorsa, D. M., Potegal, M., & Ferris, C. F. (1990). Vasopressin in the septal area of the golden hamster controls scent marking and grooming. *Physiology and Behavior, 48,* 693–699.

Isgor, C., Kabbaj, M., Akil, H., & Watson, S. J. (2004). Delayed effects of chronic variable stress during peripubertal-juvenile period on hippocampal morphology and on cognitive and stress axis functions in rats. *Hippocampus, 14,* 636–648.

Jacobsen, L. K., Krystal, J. H., Mencl, W. E., Westerveld, M., Frost, S. J., & Pugh, K. R. (2005). Effects of smoking and smoking abstinence on cognition in adolescent tobacco smokers. *Biological Psychiatry, 57,* 56–66.

Jacobus, J., Bava, S., Cohen-Zion, M., Mahmood, O., & Tapert, S. F. (2009). Functional consequences of marijuana use in adolescents. *Pharmacology, Biochemistry and Behavior, 92,* 559–565.

Jang, M.-H., Shin, M.-C., Jung, S.-B., Lee, T.-H., Bahn, G.-H., Kwon, Y. K., . . . Kim, C.-J. (2002). Alcohol and nicotine reduce cell proliferation and enhance apoptosis in dentate gyrus. *Neuroreport, 13,* 1509–1513.

Jennes, L., Dalati, B., & Conn, P. M. (1988). Distribution of gonadrotropin releasing hormone agonist binding sites in the rat central nervous system. *Brain Research, 452,* 156–164.

Jiang, W., Zhang, Y., Xiao, L., van Cleemput, J., Ji, S.-P., Bai, G., & Zhang, X. (2005). Cannabinoids promote embryonic and adult hippocampus neurogenesis and produce anxiolytic- and antidepressant-like effects. *Journal of Clinical Investigation, 115,* 3104–3116.

Johnston, L. D., O'Malley, P. M., Bachman, J. G., & Schulenberg, J. E. (2008). *Monitoring the future national results on adolescent drug use: Overview of key findings.* Bethesda, MD: National Institute on Drug Abuse.

Johnston, R. E., & Coplin, B. (1979). Development of responses to vaginal secretion and other substances in golden hamsters. *Behavioral and Neural Biology, 25,* 473–489.

Jones, D. G. (1988). Influence of ethanol on neuronal and synaptic maturation in the central nervous system-morphological investigations. *Progress in Neurobiology, 31,* 171–197.

Jones, O. D., Bonnie, R. J., Casey, B. J., Davis, A., Faigman, D. L., Hoffman, M., . . . Yaffe, G. (2014). Law and neuroscience: Recommendations submitted to the President's Bioethics Commission. *Journal of Law and the Biosciences, 1,* 224–236.

Juraska, J. M., & Markham, J. A. (2004). The cellular basis for volume changes in the rat cortex during puberty: White and gray matter. *Annals of the New York Academy of Sciences, 1021,* 431–435.

Kagan, J. (2016). An overly permissive extension. *Perspectives on Psychological Science, 11,* 442–450.

Kanayama, G., Hudson, J. I., & Pope, H. G., Jr. (2010). Illicit anabolic-androgenic steroid use. *Hormones and Behavior, 58,* 111–121.

Kaplowitz, P. B. (2008). Link between body fat and the timing of puberty. *Pediatrics, 121,* S208–S217.

Kaplowitz, P. B., Slora, E. J., Wasserman, R. C., Pedlow, S. E., & Herman-Giddens, M. E. (2001). Earlier onset of puberty in girls: Relation to increased body mass index and race. *Pediatrics, 108,* 347–353.

Kasza, K. A., Ambrose, B. K., Conway, K. P., Borek, N., Taylor, K., Goniewicz, M. L., . . . Hyland, A. J. (2017). Tobacco-product use by adults and youths in the United States in 2013–2014. *New England Journal of Medicine, 376,* 342–353.

Kellogg, C. K., & Lundin, A. (1999). Brain androgen-inducible aromatase is critical for adolescent organization of environment-specific social interaction in male rats. *Hormones and Behavior, 35,* 155–162.

Kennedy, G. C., & Mitra, J. (1963). Body weight and food intake as initiating factors for puberty in the rat. *Journal of Physiology, 166,* 408–418.

Kercmar, J., Snoj, T., Tobet, S. A., & Majdic, G. (2014). Gonadectomy prior to puberty decreases normal parental behavior in adult mice. *Hormones and Behavior, 66,* 667–673.

Kershaw, E. E., & Flier, J. S. (2004). Adipose tissue as an endocrine organ. *Journal of Clinical Endocrinology and Metabolism, 89,* 2548–2556.

Kessler, R. C., Berglund, P., Demler, O., Jin, R., Merikangas, K. R., & Walters, E. E. (2005). Lifetime prevalence and age-of-onset distributions of DSM-IV disorders in the national comorbidity survey replication. *Archives of General Psychiatry, 62,* 593–602.

Kessler, R. C., McGonagle, K. A., Zhao, S., Nelson, C. B., Hughes, M., Eshleman, S., . . . Kendler, K. S. (1994). Lifetime and 12-month prevalence of DSM-III-R psychiatric disorders in the United States. *Archives of General Psychiatry, 51,* 8–19.

Kilford, E. J., Garrett, E., & Blakemore, S.-J. (2016). The development of social cognition in adolescence: An integrated perspective. *Neuroscience and Biobehavioral Reviews, 70,* 106–120.

Kim, Y.-P., Kim, H., Shin, M.-S., Chang, H.-K., Jang, M.-H., Shin, M.-C., . . . Kim, C.-J. (2004). Age-dependence of the effect of treadmill exercise on cell proliferation in the dentate gyrus of rats. *Neuroscience Letters, 355,* 152–154.

King, J. C., Anthony, E. L. P., Fitzgerald, D. M., & Stopa, E. G. (1985). Luteinizing hormone-releasing hormone neurons in human preoptic/hypothalamus: Differential intraneural localization of immunoreactive forms. *Journal of Clinical Endocrinology and Metabolism, 60,* 88–97.

Klump, K. L. (2013). Puberty as a critical risk period of eating disorders: A review of human and animal studies. *Hormones and Behavior, 64,* 399–410.

Kodama, M., Fujioka, T., & Duman, R. S. (2004). Chronic olanzapine or fluoxetine administration increases cell proliferation in hippocampus and prefrontal cortex of adult rat. *Biological Psychiatry, 56,* 570–580.

Kokoeva, M. V., Yin, H., & Flier, J. S. (2005). Neurogenesis in the hypothalamus of adult mice: Potential role in energy balance. *Science, 310,* 679–683.

Kokoeva, M. V., Yin, H., & Flier, J. S. (2007). Evidence for constitutive neural cell proliferation in the adult murine hypothalamus. *Journal of Comparative Neurology, 505,* 209–220.

Kolb, B., Gorny, G., Limebeer, C. L., & Parker, L. A. (2006). Chronic treatment with d-9-tetrahydrocannabinol alters the structure of neurons in the nucleus accumbens shell and medial prefrontal cortex of rats. *Synapse, 60,* 429–436.

Kollins, S. H. (2008). ADHD, substance use disorders, and psychostimulant treatment. *Journal of Attention Disorders, 12,* 115–125.

Koss, W. A., Lloyd, M. M., Sadowski, R. N., Wise, L. M., & Juraska, J. M. (2015). Gonadectomy before puberty increases the number of neurons and glia in the medial prefrontal cortex of female, but not male, rats. *Developmental Psychobiology, 57,* 305–312.

Kundu, P., Benson, B. E., Rosen, D., Frangou, S., Leibenluft, E., Luh, W.-M., . . . Ernst, M. (2018). The integration of functional brain activity from adolescence to adulthood. *Journal of Neuroscience, 38,* 3559–3570.

Ladouceur, C. D., Peper, J. S., Crone, E. A., & Dahl, R. E. (2012). White matter development in adolescence: The influence of puberty and implications for affective disorders. *Developmental Cognitive Neuroscience, 2,* 36–54.

Lagace, D. C., Yee, J. K., Bolanos, C. A., & Eisch, A. J. (2006). Juvenile administration of methylphenidate attenuates adult hippocampal neurogenesis. *Biological Psychiatry, 60,* 1121–1130.

LaRoche, R. B., & Morgan, R. E. (2007). Adolescent fluoxetine exposure produces enduring, sex-specific alterations of visual discrimination and attention in rats. *Neurotoxicology and Teratology, 29,* 96–107.

Lawston, J., Borella, A., Robinson, J. K., & Whitaker-Asmitia, P. M. (2000). Changes in hippocampal morphology following chronic treatment with the synthetic cannabinoid WIN 55,212-2. *Brain Research, 877,* 407–410.

Lebel, C., & Beaulieu, C. (2011). Longitudinal development of human brain wiring continues from childhood into adulthood. *Journal of Neuroscience, 31,* 10937–10947.

LeBlanc-Duchin, D., & Taukulis, H. K. (2007). Chronic oral methylphenidate administration to periadolescent rats yield prolonged impairment of memory for objects. *Neurobiology of Learning and Memory, 88,* 312–320.

Lee, F. S., Heimer, H., Giedd, J. N., Lein, E. S., Sestan, N., Weinberger, D. R., & Casey, B. J. (2014). Adolescent mental health—opportunity and obligation. *Science, 346,* 547–549.

Lee, J.-H., Miele, M. E., Hicks, D. J., Phillips, K. K., Trent, J. M., Weissman, B. E., & Welch, D. R. (1996). Kiss-1, a novel human malignant melanoma metastasis-suppressor gene. *Journal of the National Cancer Institute, 88,* 1731–1737.

Lee, T. T., Wainwright, S. R., Hill, M. N., Galea, L. A. M., & Gorzalka, B. B. (2014). Sex, drugs, and adult neurogenesis: Sex-dependent effects of escalating adolescent cannabinoid exposure on adult hippocampal neurogenesis, stress reactivity, and amphetamine sensitization. *Hippocampus, 24,* 280–292.

Lee, Y., & Styne, D. (2013). Influences on the onset and tempo of puberty in human beings and implications for adolescent psychological development. *Hormones and Behavior, 64,* 250–261.

Lein, E., Hawrylycz, M. J., Ao, N., Ayres, M., Bensinger, A., Bernard, A., . . . Jones, A. R. (2007). Genome-wide atlas of gene expression in the adult mouse brain. *Nature, 445,* 168–176.

Lenroot, R. K., & Giedd, J. N. (2006). Brain development in children and adolescents: Insights from anatomical magnetic resonance imaging. *Neuroscience and Biobehavioral Reviews, 30,* 718–729.

Lenroot, R. K., & Giedd, J. N. (2010). Sex differences in the adolescent brain. *Brain and Cognition, 72,* 46–55.

Lerch, J. P., Worsley, K., Shaw, W. P., Greenstein, D. K., Lenroot, R. K., Giedd, J. N., & Evans, A. C. (2006). Mapping anatomical correlations across cerebral cortex (MACACC) using cortical thickness from MRI. *NeuroImage, 31,* 993–1003.

Leuner, B., Gould, E., & Shors, T. J. (2006). Is there a link between adult neurogenesis and learning? *Hippocampus, 16,* 216–224.

Leussis, M. P., & Andersen, S. L. (2008). Is adolescence a sensitive period for depression? Behavioral and neuroanatomical findings form a social stress model. *Synapse, 62,* 22–30.

Leussis, M. P., Lawson, K., Stone, K., & Andersen, S. L. (2008). The enduring effects of an adolescent social stressor on synaptic density, Part II: Poststress reversal of synaptic loss in the cortex by adinazolam and MK-801. *Synapse, 62,* 185–192.

Lewis, D. A. (2000). Schizophrenia and peripubertal refinements in prefrontal cortical circuitry. In J.-P. Bourguignon & T. M. Plant, (Eds.), *The onset of puberty in perspective* (pp. 165–177). Amsterdam, The Netherlands: Elsevier.

Li, Q., Wilson, W. A., & Swartzwelder, H. S. (2002). Differential effect of ethanol on NMDA EPSCs in pyramidal cells in the posterior cingulate cortex of juvenile and adult rats. *Journal of Neurophysiology, 87,* 705–711.

Li, W., Liu, Q., Deng, X., Chen, Y., Liu, S., & Story, M. (2017). Association between obesity and puberty timing: A systematic review and meta-analysis. *International Journal of Environmental Research and Public Health, 14,* E1266.

Lighthall, N. R., Mather, M., & Gorlick, M. A. (2009). Acute stress increases sex differences in risk seeking in the balloon analogue risk task. *PLOS ONE, 4,* e6002.

Liston, C., McEwen, B. S., & Casey, B. J. (2009). Psychosocial stress reversibly disrupts prefrontal processing and attentional control. *Proceedings of the National Academy of Sciences, 106,* 912–917.

Liston, C., Miller, M. M., Goldwater, D. S., Radley, J. J., Rocher, A. B., Hof, P. R., . . . McEwen, B. S. (2006). Stress-induced alterations in frontal cortical dendritic morphology predict selective impairments in perceptual attentional set-shifting. *Journal of Neuroscience, 26,* 7870–7874.

Logue, S., Chein, J., Gould, T., Holliday, E., & Steinberg, L. (2014). Adolescent mice, unlike adults, consume more alcohol in the presence of peers than alone. *Developmental Science, 17,* 79–85.

Lomniczi, A., Loche, A., Castellano, J. M., Ronnekleiv, O. K., Bosch, M., Kaidar, G., . . . Ojeda, S. R. (2013). Epigenetic control of female puberty. *Nature Neuroscience, 16,* 281–289.

Lomniczi, A., Wright, H., & Ojeda, S. R. (2015). Epigenetic regulation of female puberty. *Frontiers in Neuroendocrinology, 36,* 90–107.

Lopez-Larson, M. P., Bogorodzki, P., Rogowska, J., McGlade, E., King, J. B., Terry, J., & Yurgelun-Todd, D. (2011). Altered prefrontal and insular cortical thickness in adolescent marijuana users. *Behavioural Brain Research, 220,* 164–172.

Lukkes, J. L., Norman, K. J., Meda, S., & Andersen, S. L. (2016). Sex differences in the ontogeny of CRF receptors during adolescent development in the dorsal raphe nucleus and ventral tegmental area. *Synapse, 70,* 126–133.

Lumia, A. R., & McGinnis, M. Y. (2010). Impact of anabolic androgenic steroids on adolescent males. *Physiology and Behavior, 100,* 199–204.

Luna, B., Garver, K. E., Urban, T. A., Lazar, N. A., & Sweeney, J. A. (2004). Maturation of cognitive processes from late childhood to adulthood. *Child Development, 75,* 1357–1372.

Lupien, S. J., McEwen, B. S., Gunnar, M. R., & Heim, C. (2009). Effects of stress throughout the lifespan on the brain, behaviour and cognition. *Nature Reviews Neuroscience, 10,* 434–445.

Lynch, W. J. (2009). Sex and ovarian hormones influence vulnerability and motivation for nicotine during adolescence in rats. *Pharmacology, Biochemistry and Behavior, 94,* 43–50.

Magarinos, A. M., & McEwen, B. S. (1995a). Stress-induced atrophy of apical dendrites of hippocampal CA3c neurons: Comparison of stressors. *Neuroscience, 69,* 83–88.

Magarinos, A. M., & McEwen, B. S. (1995b). Stress-induced atrophy of apical dendrites of hippocampal CA3c neurons: Involvement of glucocorticoid secretion and excitatory amino acid receptors. *Neuroscience, 69,* 89–98.

Maguire, E. A., Burgess, N., & O'Keefe, J. (1999). Human spatial navigation: Cognitive maps, sexual dimorphism, and neural substrates. *Current Opinions in Neurobiology, 9,* 171–177.

Mak, G. K., Enwere, E. K., Gregg, C., Pakarainen, T., Poutanen, M., Huhtaniemi, I., & Weiss, S. (2007). Male pheromone-stimulated neurogenesis in the adult female brain: Possible role in mating behavior. *Nature Neuroscience, 10,* 1003–1011.

Malberg, J. E., Eisch, A. J., Nestler, E. J., & Duman, R. S. (2000). Chronic antidepressant treatment increases neurogenesis in adult rat hippocampus. *Journal of Neuroscience, 20,* 9104–9110.

Malone, D. T., Hill, M. N., & Rubin, R. T. (2010). Adolescent cannabis use and psychosis: Epidemiology and neurodevelopmental models. *British Journal of Pharmacology, 160,* 511–522.

Maness, P. F., & Schachner, M. (2007). Neural recognition molecules of the immunoglobulin superfamily: Signaling transducers of axon guidance and neuronal migration. *Nature Neuroscience, 10,* 19–26.

Manitt, C., Mimee, A., Eng, C., Pokinko, M., Stroh, T., Cooper, H. M., . . . Flores, C. (2011). The netrin receptor DCC is required in the pubertal organization of mesocortical dopamine circuitry. *Journal of Neuroscience, 31,* 8381–8394.

Mann, D. R., Gould, K. G., & Collins, D. C. (1984). Influence of continuous gonadotropin-releasing hormone (GnRH) agonist treatment on luteinizing hormone and testosterone secretion, the response to GnRH, and the testicular response to human chorionic gonadotropin in male rhesus monkeys. *Journal of Clinical Endocrinology and Metabolism, 58,* 262–267.

Mantzoros, C. S., Flier, J. S., & Rogol, A. D. (1997). A longitudinal assessment of hormonal and physical alterations during normal puberty in boys. V. Rising leptin levels may signal the onset of puberty. *Journal of Clinical Endocrinology and Metabolism, 82,* 1066–1070.

Maren, S., & Baudry, M. (1995). Properties and mechanisms of long-term synaptic plasticity in the mammalian brain: Relationships to learning and memory. *Neurobiology of Learning and Memory, 63,* 1–18.

Markham, J. A., Morris, J. R., & Juraska, J. M. (2007). Neuron number decreases in the rat ventral, but not dorsal, medial prefrontal cortex between adolescence and adulthood. *Neuroscience, 144,* 961–968.

Markwiese, B. J., Acheson, S. K., Levin, E. D., Wilson, W. A., & Swartzwelder, H. S. (1998). Differential effects of ethanol on memory in adolescent and adult rats. *Alcoholism: Clinical and Experimental Research, 22,* 416–421.

Marshall, W. A., & Tanner, J. M. (1969). Variations in pattern of pubertal changes in girls. *Archives of Disease in Childhood, 44,* 291–303.

Marshall, W. A., & Tanner, J. M. (1970). Variations in the pattern of pubertal changes in boys. *Archives of Disease in Childhood, 45,* 13–23.

Martin-Santos, R., Fagundo, A. B., Crippa, J. A., Atakan, Z., Bhattacharyya, S., Allen, P., . . . McGuire, P. (2010). Neuroimaging in cannabis use: A systematic review of the literature. *Psychological Medicine, 40*, 383–398.

Masten, A. (1987). Toward a developmental psychopathology of early adolescence. In M. Levin & E. McArnarny (Eds.), *Early adolescent transitions* (pp. 261–278). Lexington, KY: Heath.

Matkovic, V., Ilich, J.Z., Skugor, M., Badenhop, N.E., Goel, P., Clairmont, A., . . . Landoll, J. D. (1997). Leptin is inversely related to age at menarche in human females. *Journal of Clinical Endocrinology and Metabolism, 82*, 3239–3245.

Mattson, S. N., & Riley, E. P. (1998). A review of the neurobehavioral deficits in children with fetal alcohol syndrome or prenatal exposure to alcohol. *Alcoholism: Clinical and Experimental Research, 22*, 279–294.

McCormick, C. M., & Mathews, I. Z. (2007). HPA function in adolescence: Role of sex hormones in its regulation and the enduring consequences of exposure to stressors. *Pharmacology, Biochemistry, and Behavior, 86*, 220–233.

McCormick, C. M., & Mathews, I. Z. (2010). Adolescent development, hypothalamic-pituitary-adrenal function, and programming of adult learning and memory. *Progress in Neuro-Psychopharmacology & Biological Psychiatry, 34*, 756–765.

McCormick, C. M., Mathews, I. Z., Thomas, C., & Waters, P. (2010). Investigations of HPA function and the enduring consequences of stressors in adolescence in animal models. *Brain and Cognition, 72*, 73–85.

McCullen, P. A., Saint-Cyr, J. A., & Carlen, P. L. (1984). Morphological alterations in rat CA1 hippocampal pyramidal cell dendrites resulting from chronic ethanol consumption and withdrawal. *Journal of Comparative Neurology, 225*, 111–118.

McDonald, C. G., Dailey, V. K., Bergstrom, H. C., Wheeler, T. L., Eppolito, A. K., Smith, L. N., & Smith, R. F. (2005). Periadolescent nicotine administration produces enduring changes in dendritic morphology of medium spiny neurons from nucleus accumbens. *Neuroscience Letters, 385*, 163–167.

McDonald, C. G., Eppolito, A. K., Brielmaier, J. M., Smith, L. N., Bergstrom, H. C., Lawhead, M. R., & Smith, R. F. (2007). Evidence for elevated nicotine-induced structural plasticity in nucleus accumbens of adolescent rats. *Brain Research, 1151*, 211–218.

McDonald, H. Y., & Wojtowicz, J. M. (2005). Dynamics of neurogenesis in the dentate gyrus of adult rats. *Neuroscience Letters, 385*, 70–75.

McEwen, B. S. (1999). Stress and hippocampal synaptic plasticity. *Annual Review of Neuroscience, 22*, 105–122.

McEwen, B. S. (2005). Glucocorticoids, depression, and mood disorders: Structural remodeling in the brain. *Metabolism Clinical and Experimental, 54*, 20–23.

McEwen, B. S. (2012). The ever-changing brain: Cellular and molecular mechanisms for the effects of stressful experiences. *Developmental Neurobiology, 72*, 878–890.

McEwen, B. S., & Margarinos, A. M. (1997). Stress effects on morphology and function of the hippocampus. *Annals of the New York Academy of Sciences, 821*, 271–284.

McEwen, B. S., & McEwen, C. A. (2016). Response to Jerome Kagan's essay on stress. *Perspectives on Psychological Science, 11*, 451–455.

McIntyre, C. K., McGaugh, J. L., & Williams, C. L. (2012). Interacting brain systems modulate memory consolidation. *Neuroscience and Biobehavioral Reviews, 36*, 1750–1762.

McNay, D. E., Briancon, N., Kokoeva, M. V., Maratos-Flier, E., & Flier, J. S. (2012). Remodeling of the arcuate nucleus energy-balance circuit is inhibited in obese mice. *Journal of Clinical Investigation, 122*, 142–152.

Mechoulam, R. (1970). Marihuana chemistry. *Science, 168,* 1159–1165.

Meek, L. R., Romeo, R. D., Novak, C. M., & Sisk, C. L. (1997). Actions of testosterone in prepubertal and postpubertal male hamsters: Dissociation of effects on reproductive behavior and brain androgen receptor immunoreactivity. *Hormones and Behavior, 31,* 75–88.

Melloni, R. H., Jr., & Ricci, L. A. (2010). Adolescent exposure to anabolic/androgenic steroids and the neurobiology of offensive aggression: A hypothalamic neural model based on findings in pubertal Syrian hamsters. *Hormones and Behavior, 58,* 177–191.

Mendle, J. (2014). Beyond pubertal timing: New directions for studying individual differences in development. *Current Directions in Psychological Science, 23,* 215–219.

Mendle, J., Turkheimer, E., & Emery, R. E. (2007). Detrimental psychological outcomes associated with early pubertal timing in adolescent girls. *Developmental Review, 27,* 151–171.

Menzies, L., Goddings, A.-L., Whitaker, K. J., Blakemore, S.-J., & Viner, R. M. (2015). The effects of puberty on white matter development in boys. *Developmental Cognitive Neuroscience, 11,* 116–128.

Messina, A., Langlet, F., Chachlaki, K., Roa, J., Rasika, S., Jouy, N., . . . Prevot, V. (2016). A microRNA switch regulates the rise in hypothalamic GnRH production before puberty. *Nature Neuroscience, 19,* 835–844.

Michaud, P.-A., Suris, J.-C., & Deppen, A. (2006). Gender-related psychological and behavioural correlates of pubertal timing in a national sample of Swiss adolescents. *Molecular and Cellular Endocrinology, 254–255,* 172–178.

Miller, E. K. (2000). The prefrontal cortex and cognitive control. *Nature Reviews Neuroscience, 1,* 59–65.

Mitra, R., Jadhav, S., McEwen, B. S., Vyas, A., & Chattarji, S. (2005). Stress duration modulates the spatiotemporal patterns of spine formation in the basolateral amygdala. *Proceedings of the National Academy of Sciences, 102,* 9371–9376.

Mitra, R., & Sapolsky, R .M. (2008). Acute corticosterone treatment is sufficient to induce anxiety and amygdaloid dendritic hypertrophy. *Proceedings of the National Academy of Sciences USA, 105,* 5573–5578.

Mokrysz, C., Freeman, T. P., Korkki, K., & Curran, H. V. (2016). Are adolescents more vulnerable to the harmful effects of cannabis than adult? A placebo-controlled study in human males. *Translational Psychiatry, 6,* e961.

Mora, F., Segovia, G., & del Arco, A. (2007). Aging, plasticity and environmental enrichment: Structural changes and neurotransmitter dynamics in several areas of the brain. *Brain Research Reviews, 55,* 78–88.

Morley-Fletcher, S., Rea, M., Maccari, S., & Laviola, G. (2003). Environmental enrichment during adolescence reverses the effects of prenatal stress on play behaviour and HPA axis reactivity in rats. *European Journal of Neuroscience, 18,* 3367–3374.

Morris, S. A., Eaves, D. W., Smith, A. R., & Nixon, K. (2010). Alcohol inhibition of neurogenesis: A mechanism of hippocampal neurodegeneration in an adolescent alcohol abuse model. *Hippocampus, 20,* 596–607.

Mueller, S. C., Temple, V., Oh, E., VanRyzin, C., Williams, A., Cornwell, B., . . . Merke, D. P. (2008). Early androgen exposure modulates spatial cognition in congenital adrenal hyperplasia (CAH). *Psychoneuroendocrinology, 33,* 973–980.

Muftuler, L. T., Davis, E. P., Buss, C., Head, K., Hasso, A. N., & Sandman, C. A. (2011). Cortical and subcortical changes in typically developing preadolescent children. *Brain Research, 1399,* 15–24.

Murrin, L. C., Sanders, J. D., & Byland, D. B. (2007). Comparison of the maturation of the adrenergic and serotonergic neurotransmitter systems in the brain: Implications for differential drug effects on juveniles and adults. *Biochemical Pharmacology, 73,* 1225–1236.

Murty, V. P., Calabro, F., & Luna, B. (2016). The role of experience in adolescent cognitive development: Integration of executive, memory, and mesolimbic systems. *Neuroscience and Biobehavioral Reviews, 70,* 46–58.

Naruse, I., & Keino, H. (1995). Apoptosis in the developing CNS. *Progress in Neurobiology, 47,* 135–155.

National Institutes of Health. (2015, June 15). Consideration of sex as a biological variable in NIH-funded research (Notice no. NOT-OD-15-102). Retrieved from https://grants. nih.gov/grants/guide/notice-files/NOT-OD-15-102.html

Nelson, E. E., Leibenluft, E., McClure, E. B., & Pine, D. S. (2005). The social re-orientation of adolescence: A neuroscience perspective on the process and its relation to psychopathology. *Psychological Medicine, 35,* 163–174.

Nelson, R. J. (2011). *An introduction to behavioral endocrinology.* Sunderland, MA: Sinauer.

Newman, L. A., & McGaughy, J. (2011). Adolescent rats show cognitive rigidity in a test of attentional set shifting. *Developmental Psychobiology, 53,* 391–401.

Nixdorf-Bergweiler, B. E., Wallhausser-Franke, E., & DeVoogd, T. J. (1995). Regressive development in neuronal structure during song learning in birds. *Journal of Neurobiology, 27,* 204–215.

Novier, A., Diaz-Granados, J. L., & Matthews, D. B. (2015). Alcohol use across the lifespan: An analysis of adolescent and aged rodents and humans. *Pharmacology, Biochemistry and Behavior, 133,* 65–82.

Nunez, J. L., Lauschke, D. M., & Juraska, J. M. (2001). Cell death in the development of the posterior cortex in male and female rats. *Journal of Comparative Neurology, 436,* 32–41.

Nunez, J. L., Sodhi, J., & Juraska, J. M. (2002). Ovarian hormones after postnatal day 20 reduce neuron number in the rat primary visual cortex. *Journal of Neurobiology, 52,* 312–321.

O'Dell, L. E. (2009). A psychobiological framework of the substrates that mediate nicotine use during adolescence. *Neuropharmacology, 56,* 263–278.

Ojeda, S. R., Dubay, C., Lomniczi, A., Kaidar, G., Matagne, V., Sandau, U. S., & Dissen, G. A. (2010). Gene networks and the neuroendocrine regulation of puberty. *Molecular and Cellular Endocrinology, 324,* 3–11.

Ojeda, S. R., Lomniczi, A., Loche, A., Matagne, V., Kaidar, G., Sandau, U. S., & Dissen, G. A. (2010). The transcriptional control of female puberty. *Brain Research, 1364,* 164–174.

Ojeda, S. R., Lomniczi, A., Mastronardi, C., Heger, S., Roth, C., Parent, A.-S., . . . Mungenast, A. E. (2006). The neuroendocrine regulation of puberty: Is the time ripe for a systems biology approach? *Endocrinology, 147,* 1166–1174.

Ojeda, S. R., & Terasawa, E. (2002). Neuroendocrine regulation of puberty. In D. W. Pfaff, S. E. Fahrbach. R. T. Rubin, A. P. Arnold, & A. M. Etgen (Eds.), *Hormones, brain and behavior* (pp. 589–659). New York, NY: Elsevier.

Ojeda, S. R., & Urbanski, H. F. (1994). Puberty in the rat. In E. Knobil & J. D. Neill, (Eds.), *The physiology of reproduction* (pp. 363–409). New York, NY: Raven Press.

Oliveira-da-Silva, A., Manhaes, A. C., Cristina-Rodrigues, F., Filgueiras, C. C., & Abreu-Villaca, Y. (2010). Hippocampal increased cell death and decreased cell density elicited by nicotine and/or ethanol during adolescence are reversed during withdrawal. *Neuroscience, 167,* 163–173.

Oliveira-da-Silva, A., Vieira, F. B., Cristina-Rodrigues, F., Filgueiras, C. C., Manhaes, A. C., & Abreu-Villaca, Y. (2009). Increased apoptosis and reduced neuronal and glial densities in the hippocampus due to nicotine and ethanol exposure in adolescent mice. *International Journal of Developmental Neuroscience, 27,* 539–548.

Opendak, M., & Gould, E. (2015). Adult neurogenesis: A substrate for experience-dependent change. *Trends in Cognitive Sciences, 19,* 151–161.

Operskalski, J. T., Paul, E. J., Colom, R., Barbey, A. K., & Grafman, J. (2015). Lesion mapping of the four-factor structure of emotional intelligence. *Frontiers in Human Neuroscience, 9,* 1–11.

Packard, M. G., Cornell, A. H., & Alexander, G. M. (1997). Rewarding affective properties of intra-nucleus accumbens injections of testosterone. *Behavioral Neuroscience, 111,* 219–224.

Pajevic, S., Basser, P. J., & Fields, R. D. (2014). Role of myelin plasticity in oscillations and synchrony of neuronal activity. *Neuroscience, 276,* 135–147.

Palmer, R. H. C., Young, S. E., Hopfer, C .J., Corley, R. P., Stallings, M. C., Crowley, T. J., & Hewitt, J. K. (2009). Developmental epidemiology of drug use and abuse in adolescence and young adulthood: Evidence of generalized risk. *Drug and Alcohol Dependence, 102,* 78–87.

Pascual, M., Boix, J., Felipo, V., & Guerri, C. (2009). Repeated alcohol administration during adolescence causes changes in the mesolimbic dopaminergic and glutamatergic systems and promotes alcohol intake in the adult rat. *Journal of Neurochemistry, 108,* 920–931.

Patestas, M. A., & Gartner, L. P. (2006). *A textbook of neuroanatomy.* Oxford, England: Blackwell.

Paton, J. A., & Nottebohm, F. N. (1984). Neurons generated in the adult brain are recruited into functional circuits. *Science, 225,* 1046–1048.

Patton, G. C., & Viner, R. (2007). Pubertal transitions in health. *Lancet, 369,* 1130–1139.

Paus, T. (2010). Growth of white matter in the adolescent brain: Myelin or axon? *Brain and Cognition, 72,* 26–35.

Paus, T., Collins, D. L., Evans, A. C., Leonard, G., Pike, B., & Zijdenbos, A. (2001). Maturation of white matter in the human brain: A review of magnetic resonance studies. *Brain Research Bulletin, 54,* 255–266.

Paus, T., Zijdenbos, A., Worsley, K., Collins, D. L., Blumenthal, J., Giedd, J. N., . . . Evans, A. C. (1999). Structural maturation of neural pathways in children and adolescents: In vivo study. *Science, 283,* 1908–1911.

Pavlides, C., Nivon, L. G., & McEwen, B. S. (2002). Effects of chronic stress on hippocampal long-term potentiation. *Hippocampus, 12,* 245–257.

Payne, C., Machado, C .J., Bliwise, N. G., & Bachevalier, J. (2010). Maturation of the hippocampal formation and amygdala in *Macaca mulatta*: A volumetric magnetic resonance imaging study. *Hippocampus, 20,* 922–935.

Pazos, M. R., Nunez, E., Bentio, C., Tolon, R. M., & Romero, J. (2005). Functional neuroanatomy of the endocannabinoid system. *Pharmacology, Biochemistry and Behavior, 81,* 239–247.

Peelle, J. E., Cusack, R., & Henson, R. N. A. (2012). Adjusting for global effects in voxel-based morphometry: Gray matter decline in normal aging. *NeuroImage, 60,* 1503–1516.

Pelleymounter, M. A., Cullen, M. J., Baker, M. B., Hecht, R., Winters, D., Boone, T., & Collins, F. (1995). Effects of the *obese* gene product on body weight regulation in *ob/ob* mice. *Science, 269,* 540–543.

Penit-Soria, J., Audinat, E., & Crepel, F. (1987). Excitation of rat prefrontal cortical neurons by dopamine: An in vitro electrophysiological study. *Brain Research, 425,* 263–274.

Peper, J. S., Brouwer, R. M., Schnack, H. G., van Baal, G. C., van Leeuwen, M., van den Berg, S. M., . . . Hulshoff Pol, H. E. (2009). Sex steroids and brain structure in pubertal boys and girls. *Psychoneuroendocrinology, 34,* 332–342.

Peper, J. S., Hulshoff Pol, H. E., Crone, E. A., & van Honk, J. (2011). Sex steroids and brain structure in pubertal boys and girls: A mini-review of neuroimaging studies. *Neuroscience, 191,* 28–37.

Perrin, J. S., Herve, P.-Y., Leonard, G., Perron, M., Pike, G. B., Pitiot, A., . . . Paus, T. (2008). Growth of white matter in the adolescent brain: Role of testosterone and androgen receptor. *Journal of Neuroscience, 28,* 9519–9524.

Perry, A. N., Westenbroek, C., & Becker, J. B. (2013). Impact of pubertal and adult estradiol treatments on cocaine self-administration. *Hormones and Behavior, 64,* 573–578.

Pfeifer, J. H., Masten, C. L., Moore, W. E., Oswald, T. M., Mazziotta, J. C., Iacoboni, M., & Dapretto, M. (2011). Entering adolescence: Resistance to peer influence, risky behavior, and neural changes in emotion reactivity. *Neuron, 69,* 1029–1036.

Pham, K., Nacher, J., Hof, P. R., & McEwen, B. S. (2003). Repeated restraint stress suppresses neurogenesis and induces biphasic PSA-NCAM expression in adult rat dentate gyrus. *European Journal of Neuroscience, 17,* 879–886.

Phelps, E. A., & LeDoux, J. E. (2005). Contributions of the amygdala to emotion processing: From animal models to human behavior. *Neuron, 48,* 175–187.

Phoenix, C. H., Goy, R. W., Gerall, A. A., & Young, W. C. (1959). Organizing action of prenatally administered testosterone propionate on the tissues mediating mating behavior in the female guinea pig. *Endocrinology, 65,* 369–382.

Phuong, J., & Galvan, A. (2017). Acute stress increases risky decisions and dampens prefrontal activation among adolescent boys. *NeuroImage, 146,* 679–689.

Pian, J. P., Criado, J. R., Milner, R., & Ehlers, C. L. (2010). N-methyl-D-aspartate receptor subunit expression in adult and adolescent brain following chronic ethanol exposure. *Neuroscience, 170,* 645–654.

Piekarski, D.J ., Boivin, J. R., & Wilbrecht, L. (2017). Ovarian hormones organize the maturation of inhibitory neurotransmission in the frontal cortex at puberty onset in female mice. *Current Biology, 27,* 1735–1745.

Pierce, A. A., & Xu, A. W. (2010). De novo neurogenesis in adult hypothalamus as a compensatory mechanism to regulate energy balance. *Journal of Neuroscience, 30,* 723–730.

Pineda, R., Aguilar, E., Pinilla, L., & Tena-Sempere, M. (2010). Physiological roles of the kisspeptin/GPR54 system in the neuroendocrine control of reproduction. *Progress in Brain Research, 181,* 55–77.

Pinkston, J. W., & Lamb, R. J. (2011). Delay discounting in C57BL/6J and DBA/2J mice: Adolescent-limited and life-persistent patterns in impulsivity. *Behavioral Neuroscience, 125,* 194–201.

Pinos, H., Collado, P., Rodriguez-Zafra, M., Rodriguez, C., Segovia, S., & Guillamon, A. (2001). The development of sex differences in the locus coeruleus of the rat. *Brain Research Bulletin, 56,* 73–78.

Pope, H. G., Gruber, A. J., Hudson, J. I., Cohane, G., Huestis, M. A., & Yurgelun-Todd, D. (2003). Early-onset cannabis use and cognitive deficits: What is the nature of the association? *Drugs and Alcohol Dependence, 69,* 303–310.

Porcelli, A. J., & Delgado, M. R. (2009). Acute stress modulates risk taking in financial decision making. *Psychological Science, 20,* 278–283.

Porcelli, A. J., Lewis, A. H., & Delgado, M. R. (2012). Acute stress influences neural circuits of reward processing. *Frontiers in Neuroscience, 6,* 157.

Prendergast, B. J., Onishi, K. G., & Zucker, I. (2014). Female mice liberated for inclusion in neuroscience and biomedical research. *Neuroscience and Biobehavioral Reviews, 40,* 1–5.

Primus, R. J., & Kellogg, C. K. (1989). Pubertal-related changes influence the development of environment-related social interaction in the male rat. *Developmental Psychobiology, 22,* 633–643.

Primus, R. J., & Kellogg, C. (1990). Gonadal hormones during puberty organize environment-related social interaction in the male rat. *Hormones and Behavior, 24,* 311–323.

Primus, R. J., & Kellogg, C. K. (1991). Gonadal status and pubertal age influence the responsiveness of the benzodiazepine/GABA receptor complex to environmental challenge in male rats. *Brain Research, 561,* 299–306.

Pryce, G., & Baker, D. (2005). Emerging properties of cannabinoid medicines in management of multiple sclerosis. *Trends in Neurosciences, 28,* 272–276.

Pulsifer, M. B., Brandt, J., Salorio, C. F., Vining, E. P. G., Carson, B. S., & Freeman, J. M. (2004). The cognitive outcome of hemispherectomy in 71 children. *Epilepsia, 45,* 243–254.

Pyapali, G. K., Turner, D. A., Wilson, W. A., & Swartzwelder, H. S. (1999). Age and dose-dependent effects of ethanol on the induction of hippocampal long-term potentiation. *Alcohol, 19,* 107–111.

Quinn, H. R., Matsumoto, I., Callaghan, P. D., Long, L. E., Arnold, J. C., Gunasekaran, N., . . . McGregor, I. S. (2008). Adolescent rats find repeated d9-THC less aversive than adult rats but display greater residual cognitive deficits and changes in hippocampal protein expression following exposure. *Neuropsychopharmacology, 33,* 1113–1126.

Quiring, D. P. (1944). The transplantation of testes: As translated from Arnold Adolph Berthold original manuscript published in *Archiv fur Anatomie, Physiologie und wissenschaftliche Medicin,* pg. 42–46, 1849. *Bulletin of the History of Medicine, 16,* 399–401.

Radley, J. J., Rocher, A. B., Janssen, W. G. M., Hof, P. R., McEwen, B. S., & Morrison, J. H. (2005). Reversibility of apical dendritic retraction in the rat medial prefrontal cortex following repeated stress. *Experimental Neurology, 196,* 199–203.

Radley, J. J., Sisti, H. M., Hao, J., Rocher, A. B., McCall, T., Hof, P.R., . . . Morrison, J. H. (2004). Chronic behavioral stress induces apical dendritic reorganization of pyramidal neurons of the medial prefrontal cortex. *Neuroscience, 125,* 1–6.

Raeburn, P. (2004, October 17). Too immature for the death penalty? *The New York Times Magazine.* Retrieved from https://www.nytimes.com/2004/10/17/magazine/too-immature-for-the-death-penalty.html

Rankin, S. L., Partlow, G. D., McCurdy, R. D., Giles, E. D., & Fisher, K. R. S. (2003). Postnatal neurogenesis in the vasopressin and oxytocin-containing nucleus of the pig hypothalamus. *Brain Research, 971,* 189–196.

Raymond, A. D., Kucherapa, N. N. A., Fisher, K. R. S., Halina, W. G., & Partlow, G. D. (2006). Neurogenesis of oxytocin-containing neurons in the paraventricular nucleus (PVN) of the female pig in 3 reproductive states: Puberty gilts, adult gilts and lactating sows. *Brain Research, 1102,* 44–51.

Raznahan, A., Lerch, J. P., Lee, N., Greenstein, D., Wallace, G. L., Stockman, M., ... Giedd, J. N. (2011). Patterns of coordinated anatomical change in human cortical development: A longitudinal neuroimaging study of maturational coupling. *Neuron, 72,* 873–884.

Raznahan, A., Shaw, P. W., Lerch, J. P., Clasen, L. S., Greenstein, D., Berman, R., ... Giedd, J. N. (2014). Longitudinal four-dimensional mapping of subcortical anatomy in human development. *Proceedings of the National Academy of Sciences, 111,* 1592–1597.

Recabal, A., Caprile, T., & Garcia-Robles, M. L. A. (2017). Hypothalamic neurogenesis as an adaptive metabolic mechanism. *Frontiers in Neuroscience, 11,* 190.

Renard, J., Krebs, M.-O., Le Pen, G., & Jay, T. M. (2014). Long-term consequences of adolescent cannabinoid exposure in adult psychopathology. *Frontiers in Neuroscience, 8,* 361.

Ricci, L. A., Grimes, J. M., & Melloni, R. H., Jr. (2007). Lasting changes in neuronal activation patterns in select forebrain regions of aggressive, adolescent anabolic/androgenic steroid-treated hamsters. *Behavioural Brain Research, 176,* 344–352.

Ricci, L. A., Rasakham, K., Grimes, J. M., & Melloni, R. H., Jr. (2006). Serotonin-1A receptor activity and expression modulate adolescent anabolic/androgenic steroid-induced aggression in hamsters. *Pharmacology, Biochemistry and Behavior, 85,* 1–11.

Ricci, L. A., Schwartzer, J. J., & Melloni, R. H., Jr. (2009). Alterations in the anterior hypothalamic dopamine system in aggressive adolescent AAS-treated hamsters. *Hormones and Behavior, 55,* 348–355.

Richards, J. M., Plate, R. C., & Ernst, M. (2012). Neural systems underlying motivated behavior in adolescence: Implications for preventive medicine. *Preventive Medicine, 55,* S7–S16.

Ridderinkhof, K. R., van den Wildenberg, W. P. M., Segalowitz, S. J., & Carter, C. S. (2004). Neurocognitive mechanisms of cognitive control: The role of prefrontal cortex in action selection, response inhibition, performance monitoring, and reward-based learning. *Brain and Cognition, 56,* 129–140.

Riley, J. N., & Walker, D. W. (1978). Morphological alterations in hippocampus after long-term alcohol consumption in mice. *Science, 201,* 646–648.

Robins, S. C., Stewart, I., McNay, D. E., Taylor, V., Ciachino, C., Goetz, M., ... Placzek, M. (2013). A-tanycytes of the adult hypothalamic third ventricle include distinct populations of FGF-responsive neural progenitors. *Nature Communications, 4,* 2049.

Robinson, D. L., Zitzman, D. L., Smith, K. J., & Spear, L. P. (2011). Fast dopamine release events in the nucleus accumbens of early adolescent rats. *Neuroscience, 176,* 296–307.

Robinson, K. (1998). Implications of developmental plasticity for the language acquisition of deaf children with cochlear implants. *International Journal of Pediatric Otorhinolaryngology, 46,* 71–80.

Robson, P. (2005). Human studies of cannabinoids and medicinal cannabis. *Handbook of Experimental Pharmacology, 168,* 719–756.

Roebuck, T. M., Mattson, S. N., & Riley, E. P. (1998). A review of the neuroanatomical findings in children with fetal alcohol syndrome or prenatal exposure to alcohol. *Alcoholism: Clinical and Experimental Research, 22,* 339–344.

Rogol, A. D. (2010). Drugs of abuse and the adolescent athlete. *Italian Journal of Pediatrics, 36*, 19–24.

Romeo, R. D. (2003). Puberty: A period of both organizational and activational effects of steroid hormones on neurobehavioral development. *Journal of Neuroendocrinology, 15*, 1185–1192.

Romeo, R. D. (2010a). Adolescence: A central event in shaping stress reactivity. *Developmental Psychobiology, 52*, 244–253.

Romeo, R. D . (2010b). Pubertal maturation and programming of hypothalamic–pituitary–adrenal reactivity. *Frontiers in Neuroendocrinology, 31*, 232–240.

Romeo, R. D. (2013). The teenage brain: The stress response and the adolescent brain. *Current Directions in Psychological Science, 22*, 140–145.

Romeo, R. D. (2017). The impact of stress on the structure of the adolescent brain: Implications for adolescent mental health. *Brain Research, 1654*, 185–191.

Romeo, R. D. (2018). The metamorphosis of adolescent hormonal stress reactivity: A focus on animal models. *Frontiers in Neuroendocrinology, 49*, 43–51.

Romeo, R. D., Cook-Wiens, E., Richardson, H. N., & Sisk, C. L. (2001). Dihydrotestosterone activates sexual behavior in adult male hamsters but not in juveniles. *Physiology & Behavior, 73*, 579–584.

Romeo, R. D., Diedrich, S. L., & Sisk, C. L. (2000). Effects of gonadal steroids during pubertal development on androgen and estrogen receptor-a immunoreactivity in the hypothalamus and amygdala. *Journal of Neurobiology, 44*, 361–368.

Romeo, R. D., & McEwen, B. S. (2006). The neonatal and pubertal ontogeny of the stress response: Implications for adult physiology and behavior. In B. Arnetz & R. Ekman, (Eds.), *Stress in health and disease* (pp. 165–179). Weinheim, Germany: Wiley.

Romeo, R. D., Parfitt, D. B., Richardson, H. N., & Sisk, C. L. (1998). Pheromones elicit equivalent levels of Fos-immunoreactivity in prepubertal and adult male Syrian hamsters. *Hormones and Behavior, 34*, 48–55.

Romeo, R. D., Patel, R., Pham, L., & So, V. M. (2016). Adolescence and the ontogeny of the hormonal stress response in male and female rats and mice. *Neuroscience and Biobehavioral Reviews, 70*, 206–216.

Romeo, R. D., Wade, J., Venier, J. E., & Sisk, C. L. (1999). Androgenic regulation of hypothalamic aromatase activity in prepubertal and postpubertal male golden hamsters. *Endocrinology, 140*, 112–117.

Romeo, R. D., Wagner, C. K., Jansen, H. T., Diedrich, S. L., & Sisk, C. L. (2002). Estradiol induces hypothalamic progesterone receptors but does not activate mating behavior in male hamsters (*Mesocricetus auratus*) before puberty. *Behavioral Neuroscience, 116*, 198–205.

Roozendaal, B. (2000). Glucocorticoids and the regulation of memory consolidation. *Psychoneuroendocrinology, 25*, 213–238.

Roper v. Simmons. 543 U.S. 551 (2005).

Roth, C. L., Mastronardi, C., Lomniczi, A., Wright, H., Cabrera, R., Mungenast, A. E., . . . Ojeda, S. R. (2007). Expression of a tumor-related gene network increases in the mammalian hypothalamus at the time of female puberty. *Endocrinology, 148*, 5147–5161.

Rubino, T., & Parolaro, D. (2008). Long lasting consequences of cannabis exposure in adolescence. *Molecular and Cellular Endocrinology, 286*, S108–S113.

Rubino, T., Realini, N., Braida, D., Guidi, S., Capurro, V., Vigano, D., . . . Parolaro, D. (2009). Changes in hippocampal morphology and neuroplasticity induced by adolescent THC treatment are associated with cognitive impairment in adulthood. *Hippocampus, 19,* 763–772.

Ryback, R. S. (1973). Facilitation and inhibition of learning and memory by alcohol. *Annals of the New York Academy of Sciences, 215,* 187–194.

Rzecskowska, P. A., Hou, H., Wilson, M. D., & Palmert, M. R. (2014). Epigenetics: A new player in the regulation of mammalian puberty. *Neuroendocrinology, 99,* 139–155.

Safer, D. J., Zito, J. M., & dosReis, S. (2003). Concomitant psychotropic medication for youths. *American Journal of Psychiatry, 160,* 438–449.

Sairanen, M., Lucas, G., Ernfors, P., Castren, M., & Castren, E. (2005). Brain-derived neurotropic factor and antidepressant drugs have different but coordinated effects on neuronal turnover, proliferation, and survival in the adult dentate gyrus. *Journal of Neuroscience, 25,* 1089–1094.

Salas-Ramirez, K. Y., Montalto, P. R., & Sisk, C. L. (2008). Anabolic androgenic steroids differentially affect social behaviors in adolescent and adult male Syrian hamsters. *Hormones and Behavior, 53,* 378–385.

Salas-Ramirez, K. Y., Montalto, P. R., & Sisk, C. L. (2010). Anabolic steroids have long-lasting effects on male social behaviors. *Behavioural Brain Research, 208,* 328–335.

Sanes, J. R., & Lichtman, J. W. (1999). Development of the vertebrate neuromuscular junction. *Annual Review of Neuroscience, 22,* 389–442.

Sapolsky, R. M. (1999). Glucocorticoids, stress, and their adverse neurological effects: Relevance to aging. *Experimental Gerontology, 34,* 721–732.

Sapolsky, R. M., Krey, L. C., & McEwen, B. S. (1985). Prolonged glucocorticoid exposure reduces hippocampal neuron number: Implications for aging. *Journal of Neuroscience, 5,* 1222–1227.

Sapolsky, R. M., & Meaney, M. J. (1986). Maturation of the adrenocortical stress response: Neuroendocrine control mechanisms and the stress hyporesponsive period. *Brain Research Reviews, 396,* 64–76.

Sapolsky, R. M., Romero, L. M., & Munck, A. U. (2000). How do glucocorticoids influence stress responses? Integrating permissive, suppressive, stimulatory, and preparative actions. *Endocrine Reviews, 21,* 55–89.

Sato, S. M., Schulz, K. M., Sisk, C. L., & Wood, R. I. (2008). Adolescents and androgens, receptors and rewards. *Hormones and Behavior, 53,* 647–658.

Schaefers, A. T., Teuchert-Noodt, G., Bagorda, F., & Brummelte, S. (2009). Effect of postnatal methamphetamine trauma and adolescent methylphenidate treatment on adult hippocampal neurogenesis in gerbils. *European Journal of Pharmacology, 616,* 86–90.

Schmithorst, V. J., & Yuan, W. (2010). White matter development during adolescence as shown by diffusion MRI. *Brain and Cognition, 72,* 16–25.

Schramm-Sapyta, N. L., Cha, Y. M., Chaudhry, S., Wilson, W. A., Swartzwelder, H. S., & Kuhn, C. M. (2007). Differential anxiogenic, aversive, and locomotor effects of THC in adolescent and adult rats. *Psychopharmacology, 191,* 867–877.

Schulz, K. M., Molenda-Figueira, H. A., & Sisk, C. L. (2009). Back to the future: The organizational-activational hypothesis adapted to puberty and adolescence. *Hormones and Behavior, 55,* 597–604.

Schulz, K. M., Richardson, H. N., Zehr, J. L., Osetek, A. J., Menard, T. A., & Sisk, C. L. (2004). Gonadal hormones masculinize and defeminize reproductive behaviors during puberty in the male Syrian hamster. *Hormones and Behavior, 45,* 242–249.

Schulz, K. M., & Sisk, C. L. (2006). Pubertal hormones, the adolescent brain, and the maturation of social behaviors: Lessons from the Syrian hamster. *Molecular and Cellular Endocrinology, 254–255,* 120–126.

Schulz, K. M., & Sisk, C. L. (2016). The organizing actions of adolescent gonadal steroid hormones on brain and behavioral development. *Neuroscience and Biobehavioral Reviews, 70,* 148–158.

Schweinsburg, A. D., Schweinsburg, B. C., Medina, K. L., McQueeny, T., Brown, S. A., & Tapert, S. F. (2010). The influence of recency of use on fMRI response during spatial working memory in adolescent marijuana users. *Journal of Psychoactive Drugs, 42,* 401–412.

Scott, J. P., Stewart, J. M., & De Ghett, V. J. (1974). Critical periods in the organization of systems. *Developmental Psychobiology, 7,* 489–513.

Sebastian, C., Burnett, S., & Blakemore, S.-J. (2008). Development of the self-concept during adolescence. *Trends in Cognitive Sciences, 12,* 441–446.

Seminara, S. B., Messager, S., Chatzidaki, E. E., Thresher, R. R., Acierno, J. S., Shagoury, J. K., . . . Colledge, W. H. (2003). The *GPR54* gene as a regulator of puberty. *New England Journal of Medicine, 349,* 1614–1627.

Shannon, B. J., Raichle, M. E., Snyder, A. Z., Fair, D. A., Mills, K. L., Zhang, D., . . . Kiehl, K. A. (2011). Premotor functional connectivity predicts impulsivity in juvenile offenders. *Proceedings of the National Academy of Sciences, 108,* 11241–11245.

Shapiro, M. (2001). Plasticity, hippocampal place cells, and cognitive maps. *Archives of Neurology, 58,* 874–881.

Shaw, P., Greenstein, D., Lerch, J., Clasen, L., Lenroot, R., Gogtay, N., . . . Giedd, J. (2006). Intellectual ability and cortical development in children and adolescents. *Nature, 440,* 676–679.

Shaw, P., Kabani, N. J., Lerch, J. P., Eckstrand, K., Lenroot, R., Gogtay, N., . . . Wise, S. P. (2008). Neurodevelopmental trajectories of the human cerebral cortex. *Journal of Neuroscience, 28,* 3586–3594.

Shekhar, A., Truitt, W., Rainnie, D., & Sajdyk, T. (2005). Role of stress, corticotrophin releasing factor (CRF) and amygdala plasticity in chronic anxiety. *Stress, 8,* 209–219.

Shome, A., Sultana, R., Siddiqui, A., & Romeo, R. D. (2018). Adolescent changes in cellular proliferation in the dentate gyrus of male and female C57BL/6N mice are resilient to chronic oral corticosterone treatments. *Frontiers in Behavioral Neuroscience, 12,* 192.

Shors, T. J., Mlesegaes, G., Beylin, A., Zhao, M., Rydel, T., & Gould, E. (2001). Neurogenesis in the adult is involved in the formation of trace memories. *Nature, 410,* 372–376.

Shram, M. J., Funk, D., Li, Z., & Le, A. D. (2006). Periadolescent and adult rats respond differently in tests measuring the rewarding and aversive effects of nicotine. *Psychopharmacology, 186,* 201–208.

Shram, M .J., & Le, A. D. (2010). Adolescent male Wistar rats are more responsive than adult rats to the conditioned rewarding effects of intravenously administration nicotine in the place conditioning procedure. *Behavioural Brain Research, 206,* 240–244.

Silveri, M. M., & Spear, L. P. (1998). Decreased sensitivity to the hypnotic effects of ethanol early in ontogeny. *Alcoholism: Clinical and Experimental Research, 22,* 670–676.

Silverman, A.-J. (1976). Distribution of luteinizing hormone-releasing hormone (LHRH) in the guinea pig brain. *Endocrinology, 99,* 30–41.

Sisk, C. L. (2016). Hormone-dependent adolescent organization of socio-sexual behaviors in mammals. *Current Opinion in Neurobiology, 38,* 63–68.

Sisk, C. L., & Foster, D. L. (2004). The neural basis of puberty and adolescence. *Nature Neuroscience, 7,* 1040–1047.

Sisk, C. L., Richardson, H. N., Chappell, P. E., & Levine, L. E. (2001). In vivo gonadotropin-releasing hormone secretion in female rats during peripubertal development and on proestrus. *Endocrinology, 142,* 2929–2936.

Sisk, C. L., & Turek, F. W. (1983). Developmental time course of pubertal and photoperiodic changes in testosterone negative feedback on gonadotropin secretion in the golden hamster. *Endocrinology, 112,* 1208–1216.

Sisk, C. L., & Zehr, J. L. (2005). Pubertal hormones organize the adolescent brain and behavior. *Frontiers of Neuroendocrinology, 26,* 163–174.

Slawecki, C. J., Gilder, A., Roth, J., & Ehlers, C. L. (2003). Increased anxiety-like behavior in adult rats exposed to nicotine as adolescents. *Pharmacology, Biochemistry and Behavior, 72,* 355–361.

Smith, J. T., Acohido, B. V., Clifton, D. K., & Steiner, R. A. (2006). KiSS-1 neurones are direct targets for letpin in the *ob/ob* mouse. *Journal of Neuroendocrinology, 18,* 298–303.

Sotiras, A., Toledo, J. B., Gur, R. E., Gur, R. C., Satterthwaite, T. D., & Davatzikos, C. (2017). Patterns of coordinated cortical remodeling during adolescence and their association with functional specialization and evolution expansion. *Proceedings of the National Academy of Sciences, 114,* 3527–3532.

Sousa, N., Lukoyanov, N. V., Madeira, M. D., Almeida, O. F., & Paula-Barbosa, M. M. (2000). Reorganization of the morphology of hippocampal neurites and synapses after stress-induced damage correlates with behavioral improvement. *Neuroscience, 97,* 253–266.

Sowell, E. R., Thompson, P. M., Colin, J. H., Jernigan, T. L., & Toga, A. W. (1999). In vivo evidence for post-adolescent brain maturation in frontal and striatal regions. *Nature Neuroscience, 2,* 859–861.

Sowell, E. R., Trauner, D. A., Gamst, A., & Jernigan, T. L. (2002). Development of cortical and subcortical brain structures in childhood and adolescence: A structural MRI study. *Developmental Medicine and Child Neurology, 44,* 4–16.

Spear, L. P. (2000). The adolescent brain and age-related behavioral manifestations. *Neuroscience and Biobehavioral Reviews, 24,* 417–463.

Spear, L. P. (2009). Heightened stress responsivity and emotional reactivity during pubertal maturation: Implications for psychopathology. *Development and Psychopathology, 21,* 87–97.

Spear, L. P. (2010). *The behavioral neuroscience of adolescence.* New York, NY: Norton.

Spear, L. P., & Varlinskaya, E. I. (2010). Sensitivity to ethanol and other hedonic stimuli in an animal model of adolescence: Implications for prevention science? *Developmental Psychobiology, 52,* 236–243.

Spencer, S., & Huh, L. (2008). Outcomes of epilepsy surgery in adults and children. *Lancet Neurology, 7,* 525–537.

Squire, L. R. (1992). Memory and the hippocampus: A synthesis from findings with rats, monkeys, and humans. *Psychological Reviews, 99,* 195–231.

Staffend, N. A., Mohr, M. A., DonCarlos, L. L., & Sisk, C. L. (2014). A decrease in the addition of new cells in the nucleus accumbens and prefrontal cortex between puberty and adulthood in male rats. *Developmental Neurobiology, 74,* 633–642.

Stahl, S. M. (1992). Serotonin neuroscience discoveries usher in a new era of novel drug therapies for psychiatry. *Psychopharmacology Bulletin, 28,* 3–9.

Staiti, A. M., Morgane, P. J., Galler, J. R., Grivetti, J. Y., Bass, D. C., & Mokler, D. J. (2011). A microdialysis study of the medial prefrontal cortex of adolescent and adult rats. *Neuropharmacology, 61,* 544–549.

Starkman, M. N., Gebarski, S. S., Berent, S., & Schteingart, D. E. (1992). Hippocampal formation volume, memory dysfunction, and cortisol levels in patients with Cushing's syndrome. *Biological Psychiatry, 32,* 756–765.

Steel, R. W., Miller, J. H., Sim, D. A., & Day, D. J. (2011). Learning impairment by d(9)-tetrahydrocannabinol in adolescence is attributable to deficits in chunking. *Behavioral Pharmacology, 22,* 837–846.

Steel, R. W., Miller, J. H., Sim, D. A., & Day, D. J. (2014). Delta-9-tetrahydrocannabinol disrupts hippocampal neuroplasticity and neurogenesis in trained, but not untrained adolescent Sprague–Dawley rats. *Brain Research, 1548,* 12–19.

Steensma, T. D., Kreukels, B. P. C., de Vries, A. L. C., & Cohen-Kettenis, P. T. (2013). Gender identity development in adolescence. *Hormones and Behavior, 64,* 288–297.

Steinberg, L. (2003). Less guilty by reason of adolescence: Developmental immaturity, diminished responsibility, and the juvenile death penalty. *American Psychologist, 58,* 1009–1018.

Steinberg, L. (2009a). Adolescent development and juvenile justice. *Annual Review of Clinical Psychology, 5,* 459–485.

Steinberg, L. (2009b). Should the science of adolescent brain development inform public policy. *American Psychologist, 64,* 739–750.

Steinberg, L. (2010). A behavioral scientist looks at the science of adolescent brain development. *Brain and Cognition, 72,* 160–164.

Strang, J., Witton, J., & Hall, W. (2000). Improving the quality of the cannabis debate: Defining the different domains. *British Medical Journal, 320,* 108–110.

Stratakis, C. A., & Chrousos, G. P. (1995). Neuroendocrinology and pathophysiology of the stress system. *Annals of the New York Academy of Sciences, 771,* 1–18.

Stroud, L. R., Foster, E., Papandonatos, G. D., Handwerger, K., Granger, D. A., Kivlighan, K. T., & Niaura, R. (2009). Stress response and the adolescent transition: Performance versus peer rejection stressors. *Development and Psychopathology, 21,* 47–68.

Sturman, D. A., & Moghaddam, B. (2011). The neurobiology of adolescence: Changes in brain architecture, functional dynamics, and behavioral tendencies. *Neuroscience and Biobehavioral Reviews, 35,* 1704–1712.

Substance Abuse and Mental Health Services Administration. (2009). *Results from the 2008 National Survey on Drug Use and Health: National findings.* Rockville, MD: Author.

Suzuki, S., Oh, C., & Nakano, K. (1986). Pituitary-dependent and -independent secretion of CS caused by bacterial endotoxin in rats. *American Journal of Physiology, 250,* E470–E474.

Swartzwelder, H. S., Wilson, W. A., & Tayyeb, M. I. (1995). Differential sensitivity of NMDA receptor-mediated synaptic potentials to ethanol in immature versus mature hippocampus. *Alcoholism: Clinical and Experimental Research, 19,* 320–323.

Swithers, S. E., McCurley, M., Hamilton, E., & Doerflinger, A. (2008). Influence of ovarian hormones on development of ingestive responding to alterations in fatty acid oxidation in female rats. *Hormones and Behavior, 54,* 471–477.

Taffe, M. A., Kotzebue, R. W., Crean, R. D., Crawford, E. F., Edwards, S., & Mandyam, C. D. (2010). Long-lasting reduction in hippocampal neurogenesis by alcohol consumption in adolescent nonhuman primates. *Proceedings of the National Academy of Sciences, 107,* 11104–11109.

Tavares, M. A., Paula-Barbosa, M. M., & Gray, E. G. (1983). A morphometric Golgi analysis of the purkinje cell dendritic tree and after long-term alcohol consumption in the adult rat. *Journal of Neurocytology, 12,* 939–948.

Teicher, M. H., Andersen, S. L., & Hostetter, J. C. (1995). Evidence for dopamine receptor pruning between adolescence and adulthood in striatum but not nucleus accumbens. *Developmental Brain Research, 89,* 167–172.

Thompson, P. M., Vidal, C., Giedd, J. N., Gochman, P., Blumenthal, J., Nicolson, R., . . . Rapoport, J. (2001). Mapping adolescent brain changes reveals dynamic wave of accelerated gray matter loss in very early-onset schizophrenia. *Proceedings of the National Academy of Sciences, 98,* 11650–11655.

Toth, E., Gersner, R., Wilf-Yarkoni, A., Raizel, H., Dar, D. E., Richter-Levin, G., . . . Zangen, A. (2008). Age-dependent effects of chronic stress on brain plasticity and depressive behavior. *Journal of Neurochemistry, 107,* 522–532.

Tottenham, N., & Sheridan, M. A. (2010). A review of adversity, the amygdala and the hippocampus: A consideration of developmental timing. *Frontiers in Human Neuroscience, 3,* 1–18.

Trezza, V., Baarendse, P. J. J., & Vanderschuren, L. J. M. J. (2009). Prosocial effects of nicotine and ethanol in adolescent rats through partially dissociable neurobehavioral mechanisms. *Neuropsychopharmacology, 34,* 2560–2573.

Trezza, V., Cuomo, V., & Vanderschuren, L. J. M. J. (2008). Cannabis and the developing brain: Insights from behavior. *European Journal of Pharmacology, 585,* 441–452.

Trotman, H. D., Holtzman, C. W., Ryan, A. T., Shapiro, D. I., Macdonald, A. N., Goulding, S. M., . . . Walker, E. F. (2013). The development of psychotic disorders in adolescence: A potential role for hormones. *Hormones and Behavior, 64,* 411–419.

Tsoory, M. M., Guterman, A., & Richter-Levin, G. (2009). "Juvenile stress" alters maturation-related changes in expression of the neural cell adhesion molecule L1 in the limbic system: Relevance for stress-related psychopathologies. *Journal of Neuroscience Research, 88,* 369–380.

Turner, R .J., & Lloyd, D. A. (2004). Stress burden and the lifetime incidence of psychiatric disorder in young adults. *Archives of General Psychiatry, 61,* 481–488.

Twiggs, D. G., Popolow, H. B., & Gerall, A. A. (1978). Medial preoptic lesions and male sexual behavior: Age and environmental interactions. *Science, 200,* 1414–1415.

Urbanski, H. F., Pickle, R. L., & Ramirez, V. D. (1988). Simultaneous measurement of gonadotropin-releasing hormone, luteinizing hormone, and follicle-stimulating hormone in the orchidectomized rat. *Endocrinology, 123,* 413–419.

Uylings, H. B. M., Groenewegen, H. J., & Kolb, B. (2003). Do rats have a prefrontal cortex? *Behavioural Brain Research, 146,* 3–17.

van Amsterdam, J., Opperhuizen, A., & Hartgens, F. (2010). Adverse health effects of anabolic-androgenic steroids. *Regulatory Toxicology and Pharmacology, 57,* 117–123.

van den Bos, R., Harteveld, M., & Stoop, H. (2009). Stress and decision-making in humans: Performance is related to cortisol reactivity, albeit differently in men and women. *Psychoneuroendocrinology, 34,* 1449–1458.

van der Marel, K., Bouet, V., Meerhoff, G. F., Freret, T., Bouloudard, M., Dauphin, F., . . . Reneman, L. (2015). Effects of long-term methylphenidate treatment in adolescent and adult rats on hippocampal shape, functional connectivity, and adult neurogenesis. *Neuroscience, 309,* 243–258.

van Eerdenburg, F. J. C. M., Poot, P., Molenaar, G. J., van Leeuwen, F. W., & Swaab, D. F. (1990). A vasopressin and oxytocin containing nucleus in the pig hypothalamus that shows neural changes during puberty. *Journal of Comparative Neurology, 301,* 138–146.

Varlinskaya, E. I., & Spear, L. P. (2002). Acute effects of ethanol on social behavior of adolescent and adult rats: Role of familiarity of the test situation. *Alcoholism: Clinical and Experimental Research, 26,* 1502–1511.

Vastola, B. J., Douglas, L. A., Varlinskaya, E. I., & Spear, L. P. (2002). Nicotine-induced conditioned place preference in adolescent and adult rats. *Physiology and Behavior, 77,* 107–114.

Vaswani, M., Linda, F. K., & Ramesh, S. (2003). Role of selective serotonin reuptake inhibitors in psychiatric disorders: A comprehensive review. *Progress in Neuro-Psychopharmacology & Biological Psychiatry, 27,* 85–102.

Verdurand, M., Dalton, V .S., & Zavitsanou, K. (2010). GABAa receptor density is altered by cannabinoid treatment in the hippocampus of adult but not adolescent rats. *Brain Research, 1351,* 238–245.

Verwer, R. W., Van Vulpen, E. H., & Van Uum, J. F. (1996). Postnatal development of amygdaloid projections to the prefrontal cortex in the rat studied with retrograde and anterograde tracers. *Journal of Comparative Neurology, 376,* 75–96.

Vidal, C. N., Rapoport, J. L., Hayashi, K. M., Geaga, J. A., Sui, Y., McLemore, L. E., ... Thompson, P. M. (2006). Dynamically spreading frontal and cingulate deficits mapped in adolescents with schizophrenia. *Archives of General Psychiatry, 63,* 25–34.

Vincent, S. L., Pabreza, L., & Benes, F. M. (1995). Postnatal maturation of GABA-immunoreactive neurons of rat medial prefrontal cortex. *Journal of Comparative Neurology, 355,* 81–92.

Vining, E. P. G., Freeman, J. M., Pillas, D. J., Uematsu, S., Carson, B. S., Brandt, J. E., ... Zuckerberg, A. (1997). Why would you remove half a brain? The outcomes of 58 children after hemispherectomy—The Johns Hopkins experience: 1968–1996. *Pediatrics, 100,* 163–171.

Vogt, B. A., Finch, D. M., & Olson, C. R. (1992). Functional heterogeneity in cingulate cortex: The anterior executive and posterior evaluative regions. *Cerebral Cortex, 2,* 435–443.

Volkow, N. D., Ding, Y.-S., Fowler, J. S., Wang, G.-J., Logan, J., Gatley, J. S., ... Wolf, A. P. (1995). Is methylphenidate like cocaine? Studies of their pharmacokinetics and distribution in the human brain. *Archives of General Psychiatry, 52,* 456–463.

Vyas, A., & Chattarji, S. (2004). Modulation of different states of anxiety-like behavior by chronic stress. *Behavioral Neuroscience, 118,* 1450–1454.

Vyas, A., Jadhav, S., & Chattarji, S. (2006). Prolonged behavioral stress enhances synaptic connectivity in the basolateral amygdala. *Neuroscience, 143,* 387–393.

Vyas, A., Mitra, R., Rao, B. S. S., & Chattarji, S. (2002). Chronic stress induces contrasting patterns of dendritic remodeling in hippocampus and amygdala neurons. *Journal of Neuroscience, 22,* 6810–6818.

Vyas, A., Pillai, A. G., & Chattarji, S. (2004). Recovery after chronic stress fails to reverse amygdaloid neuronal hypertrophy and enhanced anxiety-like behavior. *Neuroscience, 128,* 667–673.

Waes, V. V., Beverley, J., Marinelli, M., & Steiner, H. (2010). Selective serotonin reuptake inhibitor antidepressants potentiate methylphenidate (Ritalin)-induced gene regulation in the adolescent striatum. *European Journal of Neuroscience, 32,* 435–447.

Wagner, I. V., Sabin, M. A., Pfaffle, R. W., Hiemisch, A., Sergeyev, E., Korner, A., & Kiess, W. (2012). Effects of obesity on human sexual development. *Nature Reviews Endocrinology, 8,* 246–254.

Wahab, F., Atika, B., Ullah, F., Shahab, M., & Behr, R. (2018). Metabolic impact on the hypothalamic kisspeptin-Kiss1r signaling pathway. *Frontiers in Endocrinology, 9,* 123.

Wahlstrom, D., White, T., & Luciana, M. (2010). Neurobehavioral evidence for changes in dopamine system activity during adolescence. *Neuroscience and Biobehavioral Reviews, 34,* 631–648.

Wallace, G. L., Dankner, N., Kenworthy, L., Giedd, J. N., & Martin, A. (2010). Age-related temporal and parietal cortical thinning in autism spectrum disorders. *Brain, 133,* 3746–3754.

Wallen, K., & Baum, M. J. (2002). Masculinization and defeminization in altrical and percocial mammals: Comparative aspects of steroid hormone action. In D. W. Pfaff, (Ed.), *Hormones, brain, and behavior* (pp. 385–423). San Diego, CA: Elsevier.

Watanabe, G., & Terasawa, E. (1989). In vivo release of luteinizing hormone releasing hormone increases with puberty in the female rhesus monkey. *Endocrinology, 125,* 92–99.

Watanabe, Y., Gould, E., Cameron, H. A., Daniels, D. C., & McEwen, B. S. (1992). Phenytoin prevents stress- and corticosterone-induced atrophy of CA3 pyramidal neurons. *Hippocampus, 2,* 431–435.

Watanabe, Y., Gould, E., & McEwen, B. S. (1992). Stress induces atrophy of apical dendrites of hippocampal CA3 pyramidal neurons. *Brain Research, 588,* 341–345.

Weiland, B. J., Thayer, R. E., Depue, B. E., Sabbineni, A., Bryan, A .D., & Hutchison, K. E. (2015). Daily marijuana use is not associated with brain morphometric measures in adolescents or adults. *Journal of Neuroscience, 35,* 1505–1512.

Weissenborn, R., & Duka, T. (2003). Acute alcohol effects on cognitive function in social drinkers: Their relationship to drinking habits. *Psychopharmacology, 165,* 306–312.

Wellman, C. L. (2001). Dendritic reorganization in pyramidal neurons in medial prefrontal cortex after chronic corticosterone administration. *Journal of Neurobiology, 49,* 245–253.

West, C. H. K., Ritchie, J. C., & Weiss, J. M. (2010). Paroxetine-induced increase in activity of locus coeruleus neurons in adolescent rats: Implications of a countertheraputic effect of an antidepressant. *Neuropsychopharmacology, 35,* 1653–1663.

Whitaker-Asmitia, P. M. (2001). Serotonin and brain development: Role in human developmental diseases. *Brain Research Bulletin, 56,* 479–485.

White, A. M., Ghia, A. J., Levin, E. D., & Swartzwelder, H. S. (2000). Binge pattern ethanol exposure in adolescent and adult rats: Differential impact on subsequent responsiveness to ethanol. *Alcoholism: Clinical and Experimental Research, 24,* 1251–1256.

White, A. M., & Swartzwelder, H. S. (2004). Hippocampal function during adolescence: A unique target of ethanol effects. *Annals of the New York Academy of Sciences, 1021,* 206–220.

White, A. M., Truesdale, M. C., Bae, J. G., Ahmad, S., Wilson, W. A., Best, P. J., & Swartzwelder, H. S. (2002). Differential effects of ethanol on motor coordination in adolescent and adult rats. *Pharmacology, Biochemistry and Behavior, 73,* 673–677.

Whitney, C., Weis, S., Krings, T., Huber, W., Grossman, M., & Kircher, T. (2008). Task-dependent modulations of prefrontal and hippocampal activity during intrinsic word production. *Journal of Cognitive Neuroscience, 21,* 697–712.

Wierenga, L. M., Bos, M. G. N., Schreuders, E., Kamp, F., Peper, J. S., Tamnes, C. K., & Crone, E. A. (2018). Unraveling age, puberty and testosterone effects on subcortical brain development across adolescence. *Psychoneuroendocrinology, 91,* 105–114.

Wilmouth, C. E., & Spear, L. P. (2004). Adolescent and adult rats' aversion to flavors previously paired with nicotine. *Annals of the New York Academy of Sciences, 1021,* 462–464.

Wilson, W., Mathew, R., Turkington, T., Hawk, T., Coleman, R. E., & Provenzale, J. (2000). Brain morphological changes and early marijuana use: A magnetic resonance and positron emission tomography study. *Journal of Addictive Disorders, 19,* 1–22.

Witt, E. M. (2010). Research on alcohol and adolescent brain development: Opportunities and future directions. *Alcohol, 44,* 119–124.

Wood, R. I. (1998). Integration of chemosensory and hormonal input in the male Syrian hamster brain. *Annals of the New York Academy of Science, 855,* 362–372.

Wood, R. I. (2004). Reinforcing aspects of androgens. *Physiology and Behavior, 83,* 279–289.

Wood, R. I., & Newman, S. W. (1995). Integration of chemosensory and hormonal cues is essential for mating in the male Syrian hamster. *Journal of Neuroscience, 15,* 7261–7269.

Woolley, C. S., Gould, E., & McEwen, B. S. (1990). Exposure to excess glucocorticoids alters dendritic morphology of adult hippocampal pyramidal neurons. *Brain Research, 531,* 225–231.

Wright, L. D., Hebert, K. E., & Perrot-Sinal, T. S. (2008). Periadolescent stress exposure exerts long-term effects on adult stress responding and expression of prefrontal dopamine receptors in male and female rats. *Psychoneuroendocrinology, 33,* 130–142.

Wright, S. (2007). Cannabinoid-based medicines for neurological disorders-clinical evidence. *Molecular Neurobiology, 36,* 129–136.

Wyshak, G., & Frisch, R. E. (1982). Evidence for a secular trend in age of menarche. *New England Journal of Medicine, 306,* 1033–1035.

Yang, P. B., Swann, A. C., & Dafny, N. (2010). Psychostimlulants given in adolescence modulate their effects in adulthood using the open field and the wheel-running assays. *Brain Research Bulletin, 82,* 208–217.

Young, S. E., Corley, R. P., Stallings, M. C., Rhee, S. H., Crowley, T. J., & Hewitt, J. K. (2002). Substance use, abuse and dependence in adolescence: Prevalence symptom profiles and correlates. *Drug and Alcohol Dependence, 68,* 309–322.

Yurgelun-Todd, D. (2007). Emotional and cognitive changes during adolescence. *Current Opinion in Neurobiology, 17,* 251–257.

Zhang, Y., Proenca, R., Maffei, M., Barone, M., Leopold, L., & Friedman, J. M. (1994). Positional cloning of the mouse *obese* gene and its human homologue. *Nature, 372,* 425–432.

Zhao, C., Deng, W., & Gage, F. H. (2008). Mechanisms and functional implications of adult neurogenesis. *Cell, 132,* 645–660.

Zhou, F. C., Anthony, B., Dunn, K. W., Lindquist, W. B., Xu, Z. C., & Deng, P. (2007). Chronic alcohol drinking alters neuronal dendritic spines in the brain reward center nucleus accumbens. *Brain Research, 1134,* 148–161.

Zhu, N., Weedon, J., & Dow-Edwards, D. L. (2007). Oral methylphenidate improves spatial learning and memory in pre- and periadolescent rats. *Behavioral Neuroscience, 121,* 1272–1279.

Index